CRANIOFACIAL INJURIES FOR NONSPECIALISTS

CRANIOFACIAL INJURIES FOR NONSPECIALISTS

Editors

Abdulhakim Zaggut
Queen Mary University of London, UK

Sabah Kalamchi
AT Still University, USA

Muhammad Rahman
Queen Mary University of London, UK

Malcolm Harris
University College London, UK

World Scientific

NEW JERSEY · LONDON · SINGAPORE · BEIJING · SHANGHAI · HONG KONG · TAIPEI · CHENNAI · TOKYO

Published by

World Scientific Publishing Europe Ltd.

57 Shelton Street, Covent Garden, London WC2H 9HE

Head office: 5 Toh Tuck Link, Singapore 596224

USA office: 27 Warren Street, Suite 401-402, Hackensack, NJ 07601

Library of Congress Cataloging-in-Publication Data
Names: Zaggut, Abdulhakim, editor. | Kalamchi, Sabah, editor. |
 Rahman, Muhammad, editor. | Harris, Malcolm, editor.
Title: Craniofacial injuries for nonspecialists / editors, Abdulhakim Zaggut, Queen Mary
 University of London, UK, Sabah Kalamchi, AT Still University, USA, Muhammad Rahman,
 Queen Mary University of London, UK, Malcolm Harris, University College London, UK.
Description: New Jersey : World Scientific, [2022] | Includes bibliographical references and index.
Identifiers: LCCN 2021049383 | ISBN 9781800610187 (hardcover) |
 ISBN 9781800610194 (ebook) | ISBN 9781800610200 (ebook other)
Subjects: LCSH: Face--Wounds and injuries. | Skull--Wounds and injuries. |
 Face--Surgery. | Skull--Surgery.
Classification: LCC RD523 .C723 2022 | DDC 617.5/2044--dc23/eng/20211109
LC record available at https://lccn loc.gov/2021049383

British Library Cataloguing-in-Publication Data
A catalogue record for this book is available from the British Library.

For any available supplementary material, please visit
https://www.worldscientific.com/worldscibooks/10.1142/Q0299#t=suppl

Desk Editors: Soundararajan Raghuraman/Joy Quek

Typeset by Stallion Press
Email: enquiries@stallionpress.com

Editors and Contributors

Editors

Abdulhakim Zaggut BDS, MSc, PhD
Barts and The London School of Medicine and Dentistry
Queen Mary University London, UK
The Dental School, Misrata University, Libya
Oral and Maxillofacial Surgeon, Misrata Cancer Institute Hospital

Sabah Kalamchi DDS, FDSRCS
Professor and Director Oral and Maxillofacial Surgery
Arizona School of Dentistry and Oral Health, Arizona, USA
Diplomate, American Board of Oral and Maxillofacial Surgery
Fellow Faculty Royal College of Surgeons, UK

Muhammad M. Rahman PhD
Postdoctoral Research Associate
Barts and The London School of Medicine and Dentistry
Queen Mary University London, UK

Malcolm Harris DSc, MD, FRCS Edin. FDSRCS (Eng.)
Emeritus Professor Oral and Maxillofacial Surgery
University College London, London, UK

Contributors

Muhammed Aqeel Aslam BDS, MFDS RCSEd, FCPS
Assistant Professor, Oral and Maxillofacial Surgery
Muhammad Medical & Dental College, Mirpurkhas, Pakistan

Syed Mahmood Haider BDS, MSc, FFDRCS, FDCRCS, FCPS, FDSRCP
Visiting Professor in the Department of Faciomaxillary Surgery
Karachi Medical & Dental College, University of Karachi, Karachi, Pakistan
Visiting Consultant Ziauddin University Hospital, Clifton, Karachi
National Institute of Oral Diseases, Defence, Karachi, Pakistan
Navy Hospital, PNS Shifa, Karachi, Pakistan

Zia Uddin A. Kashmiri MBBS, MCPS, FCPS
Professor, Department of Anaesthesia
Dow University of Health Sciences, Karachi, Pakistan

Mohammed Sumair Khan BDS, MSc., MFDS RCPSG
Restorative & Implant Dentist
London, UK

Ian Loh FRACS, MBBS, MS, PGDip
Craniofacial Surgeon
Royal Children's Hospital, Melbourne, Australia

John H. Phillips MD, MA, B.Sc., FRCSC
Associate Professor, The Hospital for Sick Children Centre for Craniofacial Care and Research
Division of Plastic Surgery, University of Toronto, Canada

Hajra Rana BDS
Resident Medical Officer, Dept of Oral & Maxillofacial Surgery
SMBB Institute of Trauma, Karachi, Pakistan

Eran Regev DMD, MD
Professor Specialist in Oral and Maxillofacial Surgery
Senior Lecturer Faculty of Medicine, The Hebrew University
Jerusalem, Israel
Head of Oral and Maxillofacial Surgery, Shaare Zedek Medical
Centre, Jerusalem, Israel
Faculty in the AOCMF

Saad Uddin Siddiqui BDS, MFDS RCSEd, MFDS RCPSG,
MOMS RCSEd
Assistant Professor, Dow University of Health Sciences, Karachi
Pakistan

Rephael Zeltser DMD, MD
Emeritus Professor Specialist in Oral and Maxillofacial Surgery
Hadassah Hebrew University Medical Centre, Jerusalem, Israel

Contents

Introduction

'The Management of Craniofacial Injuries for Non-Specialists' was proposed by Dr Abdulhakim Zaggut as a result of his experience as a craniofacial surgeon in the Libyan civil war during the 'Arab Spring' of 2011.

The book describes and contrasts the treatment of violent craniofacial injuries in 'austere' environments and in 'wealth and peace' settings. An 'austere' environment is defined as an area with fighting, environmental hazards and an unreliable source of electricity.

The chapters feature the unique experiences of surgeons from different parts of the world, who contribute their exclusive patient cases allowing for an in-depth comparison of injuries in both types of environment. Further to this, craniofacial injuries and management are evaluated and investigated from many perspectives including training, simulation methods, radiographic imaging and post-traumatic stress disorder.

The problem of lack of resources and qualified personnel in a conflict zone inspired the development of a training programme to teach non-specialist surgeons selected craniofacial techniques which greatly improve patient outcome. The head and neck region is critical for sensory input, facial movement and communication, therefore any techniques that allow a patient a better quality of life are of the greatest priority. The careful management of soft tissue to minimise any disfigurement is also vital. This book begins with the description of a successful one day simulated training programme.

Simulation training is now well recognised as a reliable basis for training non-specialist surgeons, whether in a war zone or a 'wealth and peace' setting. A contemporary issue has been the

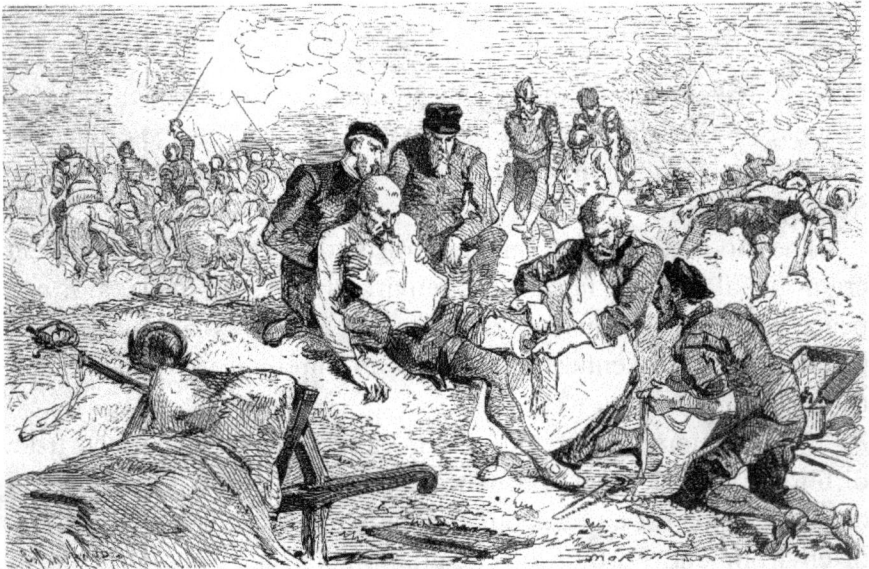

Figure 1   Ambroise Paré (1510–1590) amputating a mutilated leg

Source: https://commons.wikimedia.org/wiki/File:Ambroise_Par%C3%A9,_on_the_battlefield_using_a_ligature_for_the_a_Wellcome_L0018530.jpg#file. Credit: Wellcome Library, London. Wellcome Images images@wellcome.ac.uk http://wellcomeimages.org Ambroise Paré, on the battlefield using a ligature for the artery of an amputated leg of a soldier. Wood engraving by C. Maurand. Copyrighted work available under Creative Commons Attribution only licence CC BY 4.0 http://creativecommons.org/licenses/by/4.0/

COVID-19 pandemic which demonstrated the value of simulation training for retired medical and dental specialists, medical students, nurses and ancillaries to make good the deficiency of an overcommitted health service.

The value of simulation training contradicts the observation of 16th century surgeon Ambroise Paré that the gap between surgical training and its implementation is on the battlefield. He declared that, "He who desires to practice surgery must go to war!".

We would like to express our gratitude to: (in alphabetical order)

Habib Ellamushi MBChB, FRCS, FRCS(SN)
Consultant Neurosurgeon and Spinal Surgeon, The Royal London Hospital, London, UK

Amerigo Giudice MD, PhD
Associate Professor, Department of Health Sciences, School of Medicine and Surgery, University Magna Graecia of Catanzaro, Italy

Simon Holmes FDS RCS FRCS
Professor of Craniofacial Traumatology & Maxillofacial Surgeon, Dept Oral and Maxillofacial Surgery, Bart's and the London NHS Trust, London, UK

Eleni Aliki Nikolopoulou MBBS,
Vascular Surgeon, Basildon University Hospital, Barts and The London School of Medicine and Dentistry, London, UK

David Nott MBBS, FRCS
Consultant General Surgeon and Tutor of the RCS (Eng), Chelsea and Westminster, St Marys, Royal Marsden. London

Mohamed Shibu MBBS, FRCS (Edin), FRCS Plastic
Consultant Plastic and Reconstructive Surgeon, Bart's and Royal
London Hospital. London, UK

Tarek Youssef
Consultant Anaesthesiologist, Banner Desert medical centre, Mesa,
Arizona, USA

Noor Zaggut
Artist

Chapter 1

Simulated Craniofacial Training

Abdulhakim Zaggut, Malcolm Harris, and Muhammad M. Rahman

Introduction

Surgeons performing emergency surgery in austere environments face a number of obstacles due to the unpredictability of the environment. The primary challenge they face is the high number of casualties requiring immediate life-saving attention, and beyond this, attempting secondary procedures that can significantly improve long-term quality of life, given that it is very unlikely that patients will return for such treatment.

This one-day simulated trauma training programme for non-specialist surgeons aims to teach relatively fast craniofacial techniques with long-lasting benefits. The training programme was devised for clinicians deficient in craniofacial surgical training and designed by specialists to cover trauma training without the expense of cadavers or any risk to patients.

This chapter describes six simulation skill stations. Four of these utilised sheep's heads to teach craniotomy, epistaxis, canthotomy, cantholysis, and external pin fixation for mandibular fractures. The remaining two skill stations taught mandible fracture fixation skills using plaster dental models designed to simulate jaw fixation with the Erich arch bar and dental eyelet wiring.

The trainees were scored for each of the six skill stations and recorded using hierarchical task analysis (HTA) with the aim to improve surgical competence regardless of their medical or dental background and experience level. Furthermore, the training course was designed to use readily available and abundant materials simulating austere environment constraints. Finally, the training programme was created with the intention that it could be used to train surgeons currently situated in austere environments, without the requirement of a highly skilled demonstrator or specialist teaching models.

The programme is based on the Surgical Training Courses for Austere Environments (STAE), Royal College of Surgeons (Eng.) hosted twice a year by David Nott, an expert in war trauma (Figure 1.1).

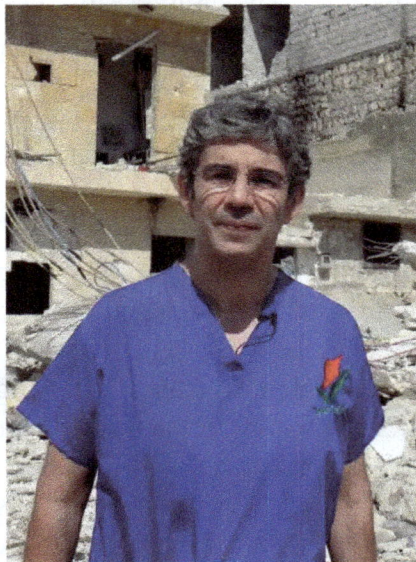

Figure 1.1   David Nott.

Source: Photograph: Channel 4/PA via *The Guardian*.

Approximately 85% of the STAE courses are spent on cadaver surgery over five days, whereas this one-day course does not use human cadavers, overcoming the problems of their lack of availability, the cost of storage, and ethical constraints.[1,2] The simulation alternatives, such as the sheep's head and plaster dental models, were used as alternative to cadavers for this one-day non-specialist course.

The Simulated Course

This course for non-specialists in a war zone would also provide appropriate training for dealing with aggression, such as an act of terrorism in an affluent and otherwise peaceful environment.

The 11 trainees participating in this course had medical or dental qualifications but no craniofacial experience.

The two demonstrators were a maxillofacial surgeon and a neurosurgeon, supported by 15 specialist assistants. The anonymised trainees filled in questionnaires to identify their level of knowledge, which included pre- and post-training checklists for each skill station. The resulting scores were evaluated by HTA which estimates how a complex task is evaluated by a measure of its components. Each skill was assessed by the specialists before and after the training, and the HTA measures of the trainees were compared statistically.

Trainees were also given health and safety instructions for using animal tissue.

Skill stations 1 to 4 used sheep's heads, while skill stations 5 and 6 utilised plaster models of the human dentition. Ethical approval for the study was obtained from the Queen Mary University London, and the programme lasted nine and a half hours (Figure 1.2).

Skill Station 1: Craniotomy Surgical Technique

Craniotomy is a vital surgical procedure for gaining access to extra- or intracranial skull fractures and intracranial haemorrhage.

Station 1
Craniotomy Surgical Technique

↓

Station 2
Nasal Packing for Epistaxis

↓

Station 3
Lateral Canthotomy and Cantholysis

↓

Station 4
External Pin Fixation for Mandibular Fractures

↓

Station 5
The Erich Arch Bar and Plaster Dental Models

↓

Station 6
Intermaxillary Fixation Using Dental Eyelet Loops

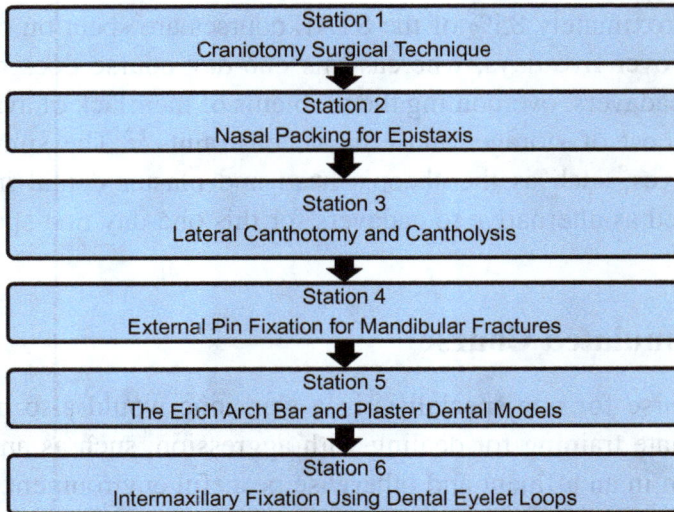

Figure 1.2   Six skill stations designed for a one-day simulated craniofacial course.

This simulated procedure requires a sheep's head and the following instruments (Figure 1.3):

(1) An electrical or manual drill.
(2) Scalpels No. 10 and No. 15.
(3) Periosteal elevator.
(4) A 10-ml syringe with 22–24G needle for saline irrigation.
(5) Fine straight arterial forceps and scissors.
(6) 4/0 polyglyconate suture or 3/0 black silk, as both have strength.

Sheep's heads can be difficult to obtain from an abattoir, and the fur removal creates burnt skin which also needs to be removed. In this example, the fur has been stripped off at the abattoir and the skin decontaminated.

An electrical surgical drill is useful to make the calvarium burr holes, but in a war environment, a manual drill or brace and bit may be necessary due to power failures.

It is important to identify the midline of the sheep's head to avoid the superior sagittal venous sinus (Figure 1.4).

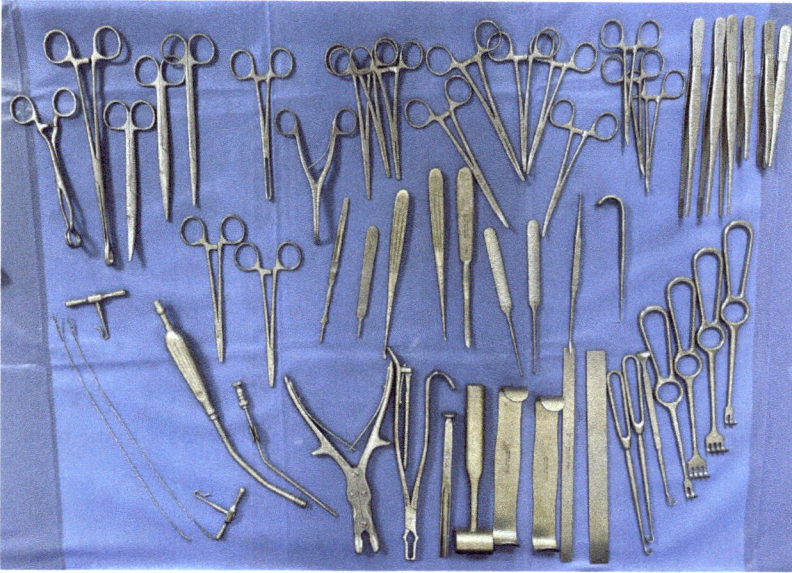

(a)

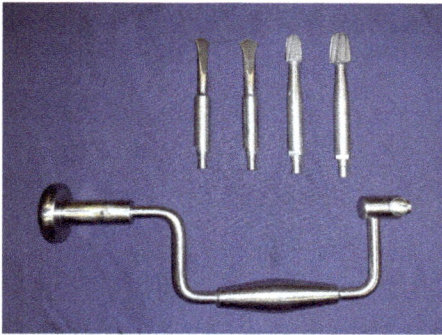

(b)

Figure 1.3   (a) Craniotomy instruments (b) a manual drill.

The craniotomy is located over the suggested site of the haematoma (Figure 1.5). Skin incisions and flaps can be S or rectangular shaped.

Multiple bone burr holes are drilled with an electrical or manual drill to outline the craniotomy (Figure 1.6), then scalpel cuts are made between the drilled holes, and the bone cortex is elevated (Figure 1.7).

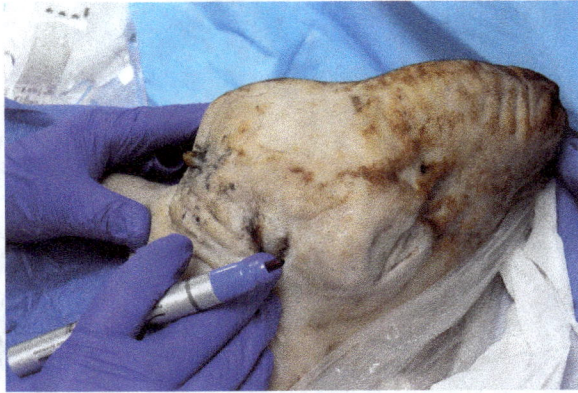

Figure 1.4 Optimal position for the sheep's head is facing to the right.

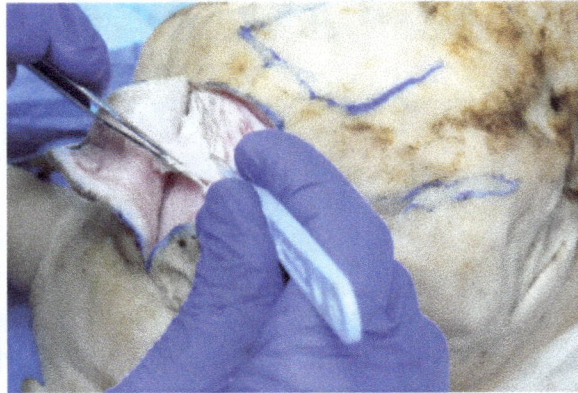

Figure 1.5 Craniotomy located over the suggested site of the haematoma.

This bone flap exposes the underlying pericranium which is carefully dissected and raised. The exposed dura is then opened using scissors to preserve the dural flap blood supply (Figure 1.8).

The brain is exposed and irrigated with normal saline, and any haematoma is identified and evacuated. The dura is now sutured if possible but can be left open if there is brain oedema. The bone flap is replaced and secured using non-resorbable sutures or miniplates.

A drain is inserted, and the skin flap is sutured.

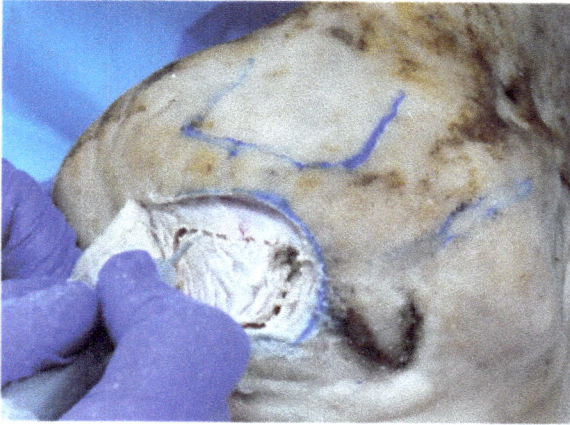

Figure 1.6 Multiple bone burr holes are drilled with an electrical or manual drill to outline the craniotomy.

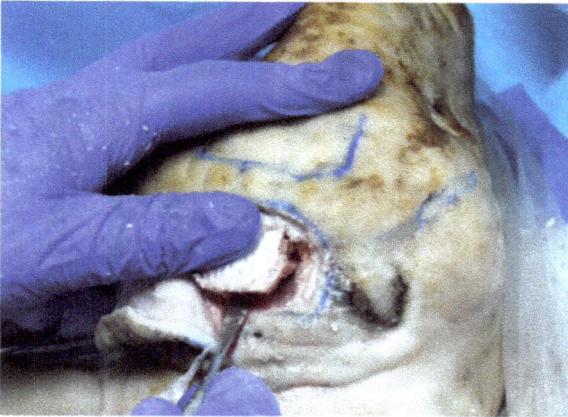

Figure 1.7 Bone cortex is elevated.

Eight steps of this surgical procedure were marked by a neuro-surgeon pre- and post-training, and HTA training results can be seen in the bar chart. The Wilcoxon signed-rank test showed that simulated craniotomy training elicited a statistically significant improvement in overall skills: a pre-training score mean of 15.9 compared to a post-training score mean of 33.2 (Z = -2.936, $p <$ 0.01). The trainee scores improved in every one of the eight steps of craniotomy training (Figure 1.9).

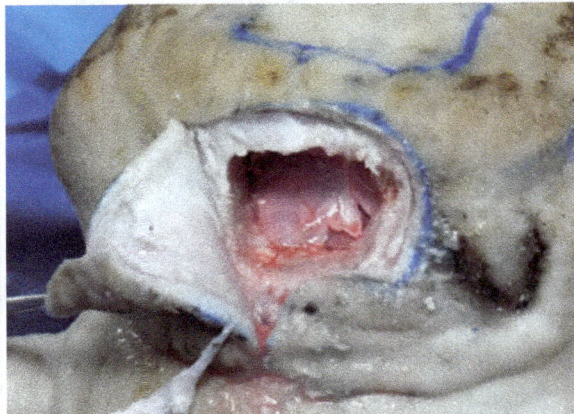

Figure 1.8   Brain is exposed.

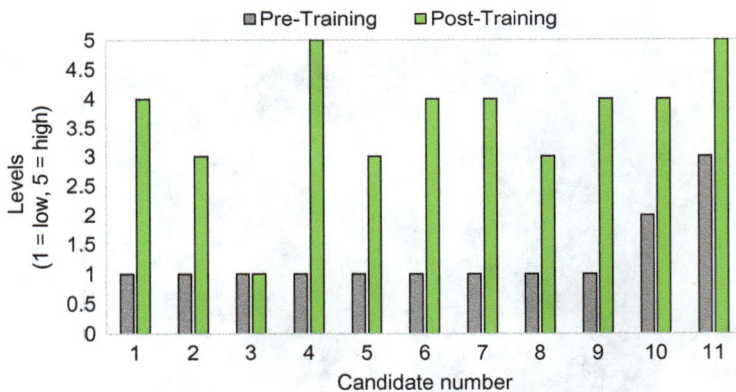

Figure 1.9   Results of each trainee showing pre- and post-training levels for craniotomy skills ($N = 11$).

Skill Station 2: Nasal Packing for Epistaxis

(Also see Chapter 2: ATLS, section on Epistaxis).

Facial trauma commonly causes epistaxis especially from the antero-inferior nasal septum (Little's area), where four arteries anastomose to form a vascular plexus which may bleed and need control (Figures 1.10 and 1.11).

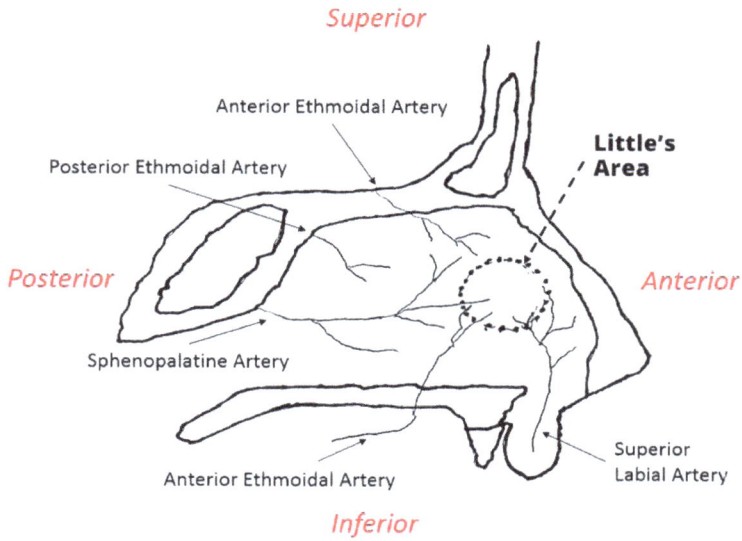

Figure 1.10   Little's area.

Source: Image licensed under CC BY-SA 4.0. By Mbuchko3.

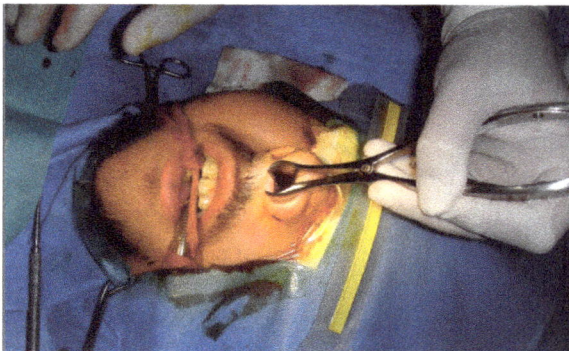

Figure 1.11   Nasal speculum or rhinoscope.

Instruments:

1. 10-ml syringe with 22–24G needle.
2. Female Foley catheter.
3. Local anaesthetic (2% lignocaine with 1/200,000 adrenaline).

4. Fine dissection forceps.
5. Straight arterial forceps and scissors.
6. Petroleum ribbon gauze.
7. Umbilical plastic clips.

An anterior bleeding point can be simply compressed or cauterised by applying silver nitrate or lidocaine (2%) with adrenaline (1/200 000) using an anterior rhinoscope; however, this cannot be demonstrated with a sheep's head.

Of primary importance is to establish if a bleeding patient is taking medication, such as anticoagulants or aspirin, or has uncontrolled hypertension.

Suction is used to remove blood clot from the nose and a local anaesthetic spray (lidocaine 2%) and adrenaline (1/200,000) for haemostasis.

Figure 1.12 shows the three methods of nasal packing:

(i) inflating the balloon of a Foley catheter;
(ii) petroleum jelly gauze packing;
(iii) both of the above, together.

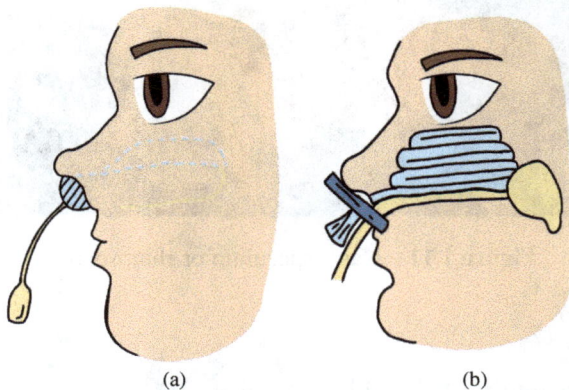

(a)   (b)

Figure 1.12   (a) Posterior packing with the Foley balloon; (b) anterior packing with petroleum jelly gauze retained by anterior umbilical clamp to protect the philtrum and nasal cartilage.

Before inserting a Foley catheter to arrest the haemorrhage, aspirate nasal clots and administer an antifibrinolytic agent to arrest the bleeding and promote haemostasis, such as tranexamic acid (TXA), epsilon-aminocaproic acid, or aprotinin (Trasylol, Bayer).

The specialist nasal catheter shown in Figure 1.13 has two balloons, one in the front and one in the back. Figure 1.14 shows how

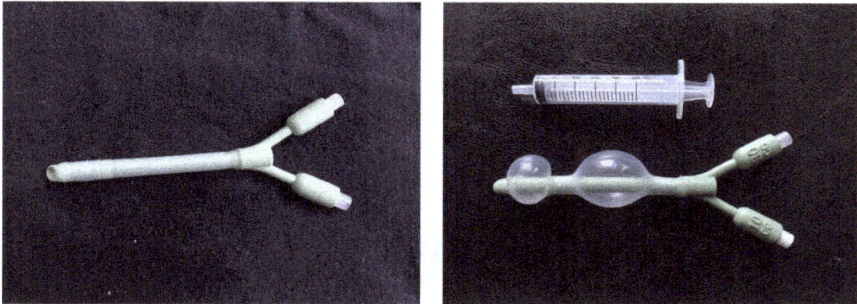

Figure 1.13 Catheter balloons are inflated with 10 ml of sterile saline or water, one anterior and one posterior.

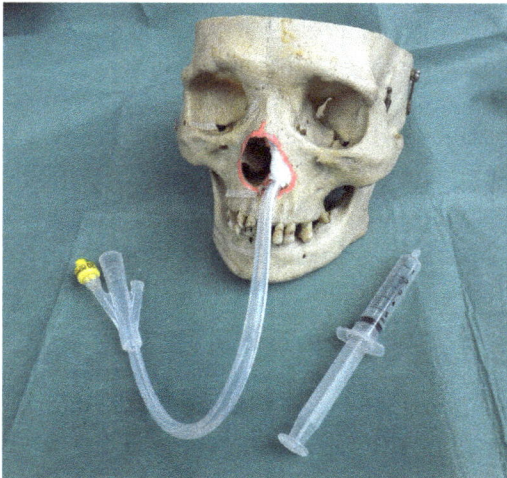

Figure 1.14 Foley catheter with single balloon, inflated with 10 ml of sterile saline or water.

in an austere environment a cheap substitute is to use the standard catheter which are plentifully available in hospitals.

With bilateral bleeding, as with a midface fracture, lubricate two catheters with petroleum jelly and insert them 10 or 12 cm into each nostril until they appear in the oropharynx (Figure 1.15).

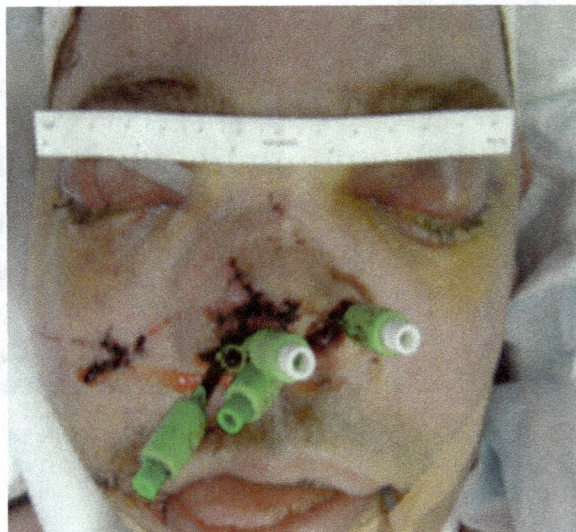

Figure 1.15 Bilateral nasal catheters in a patient with comminuted midface fractures. Attribution: Mike Perry and Simon Holmes.

However, posterior displacement of the Foley catheter balloon can compromise the airway, and if the balloon which contains water is ruptured, this can result in aspiration.

There are three steps for nasal packing to arrest a traumatic nasal haemorrhage that can be demonstrated in a sheep's head (Figures 1.16 and 1.17):

(1) The Foley catheter is inserted through the anterior nares.
(2) The catheter is positioned at the back of the nose so that when inflated, the balloon tamponades the nasopharynx and secures the catheter in place.

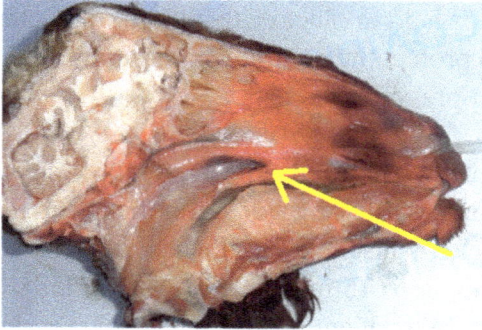

Figure 1.16   Section of the sheep's head showing the posterior inflated balloon in the nasopharynx at the posterior choanae.

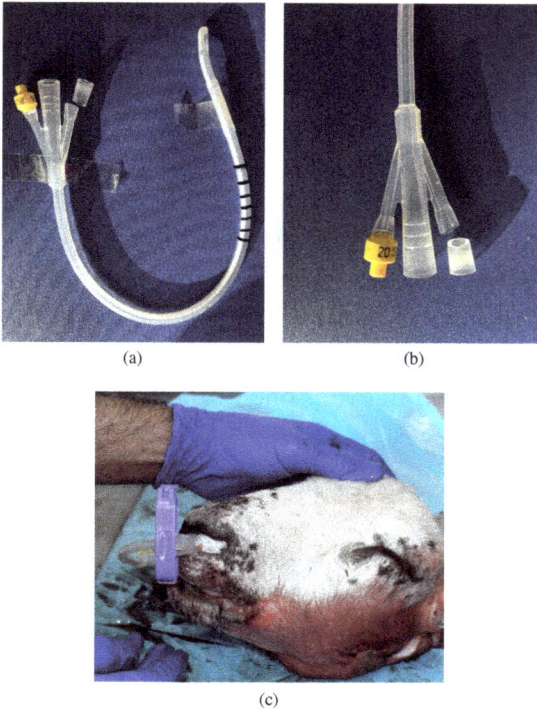

(a)

(b)

(c)

Figure 1.17   (a) The Foley catheter is marked with measurements in black ink; (b) a ring is cut from the catheter bag and slid onto the end of the catheter; (c) the anterior nasal end of the catheter is secured with a blue sealing clip clamp. The ring protects the cartilage from the pressure of the clip.

(3) The balloon is held in place with an umbilical clamp at the anterior nares to protect the columella and septum, with a soft dressing, to avoid pressure necrosis.

The sheep's head is an invaluable model for simulating nasal packing. However, the nasal floor is longer in the sheep than in a human. Ideally, the catheter is inserted into the nasopharynx area and the balloon inflated with 10 to 15 ml saline or water. This is a better option than air inflation. In a patient however, the catheter should not be left inserted for more than 48 h to avoid damage to the nasal cartilage.

Most of the trainees had no experience of nasal packing using a Foley catheter. Despite this, post-training showed bar-chart scores had improved significantly (see Figure 1.18). Six out of the 11 trainees initially failed the task which improved to one out of 11 failing post-training. The critical step for passing this task was the correct insertion of the catheter and its positioning in the nasopharynx, and all the candidates passed this in post-training with scores above 73%, with eight candidates obtaining full marks.

The Wilcoxon signed-rank test of HTA data showed that nasal packing training created a significant increase in trainee scores compared to pre-training scores ($Z = -2.94$, $p < 0.01$) with a mean post-training score of 26.5 compared to a pre-training score mean of 11.9. These scores improved in every one of the trainees (Figure 1.18).

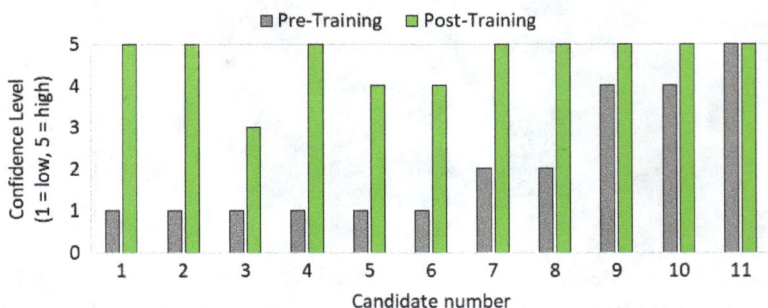

Figure 1.18   Candidates pre- and post-training results for nasal packing.

One shortcoming of this model is the lack of blood or fluid to demonstrate that the packing actually stopped the bleeding into the nasopharynx. This could be simulated with a syringe to inject a fluid dye through the nostril into the nasopharynx to determine how much could be aspirated.

Skill Station 3: Lateral Canthotomy and Cantholysis

(Also see Chapter 2, Retrobulbar haemorrhage and the orbital compartment syndrome)

Retrobulbar haemorrhage is a devastating complication associated with facial trauma. It can rapidly fill the orbit behind the globe, compressing it to cause an 'orbital compartment syndrome' which compresses the optic nerve and its vascular supply leading to permanent blindness.

Instruments:
(1) Sterile gauze gloves and drapes.
(2) 10-ml syringe with a 22–24G needle.
(3) Local anaesthetic (lignocaine 2% with adrenaline 1:200,000) for infiltration into the lateral canthus at the orbital rim to enable the cantholysis incision.
(4) Fine-toothed forceps or needle holder or haemostat, toothed forceps, and iris scissors.
(5) Straight arterial forceps and tenotomy scissors.

Each trainee was provided with three orbits with simulation of the compartment syndrome created by the post-orbital injection of glycerine and was instructed how to perform both canthotomy and cantholysis. It would have been prohibitively expensive to give each trainee three orbits from cadavers.

Their performance was video-recorded, and the assessment was made from the videos judged by two ophthalmic surgeons before and after training.

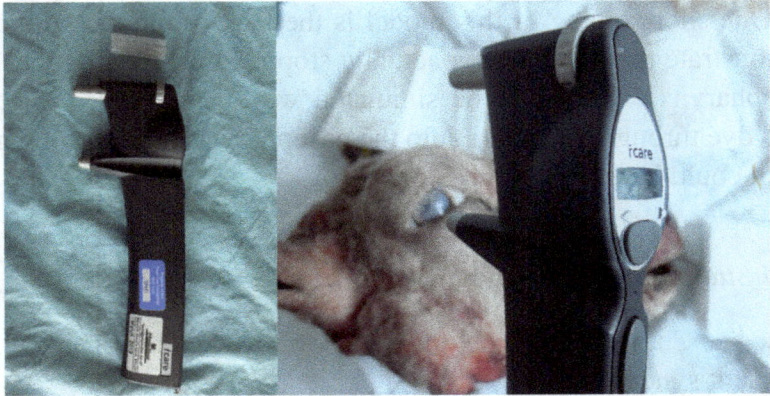

Figure 1.19   Testing intraocular pressure (IOP) using tonometry. This was not effective in the sheep's head although it works well in humans.

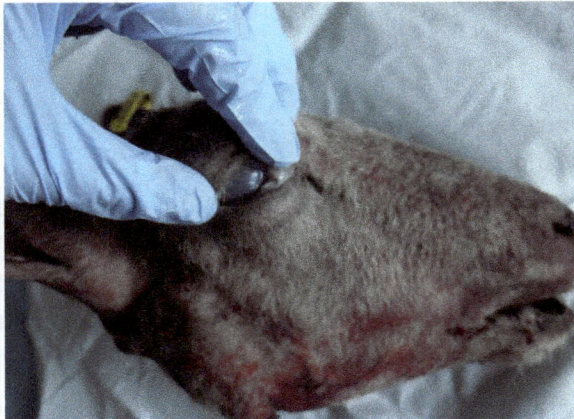

Figure 1.20   Estimation of the intraocular pressure using gloved digital compression.

Experimental canthotomy and cantholysis are divided into six tasks for evaluation (see Figures 1.19, 1.20 and 1.21):

(a) The intraocular pressure was raised by injecting saline and glycerine to simulate the retrobulbar haemorrhage. This is measured digitally by applying digital pressure on each side of the globe

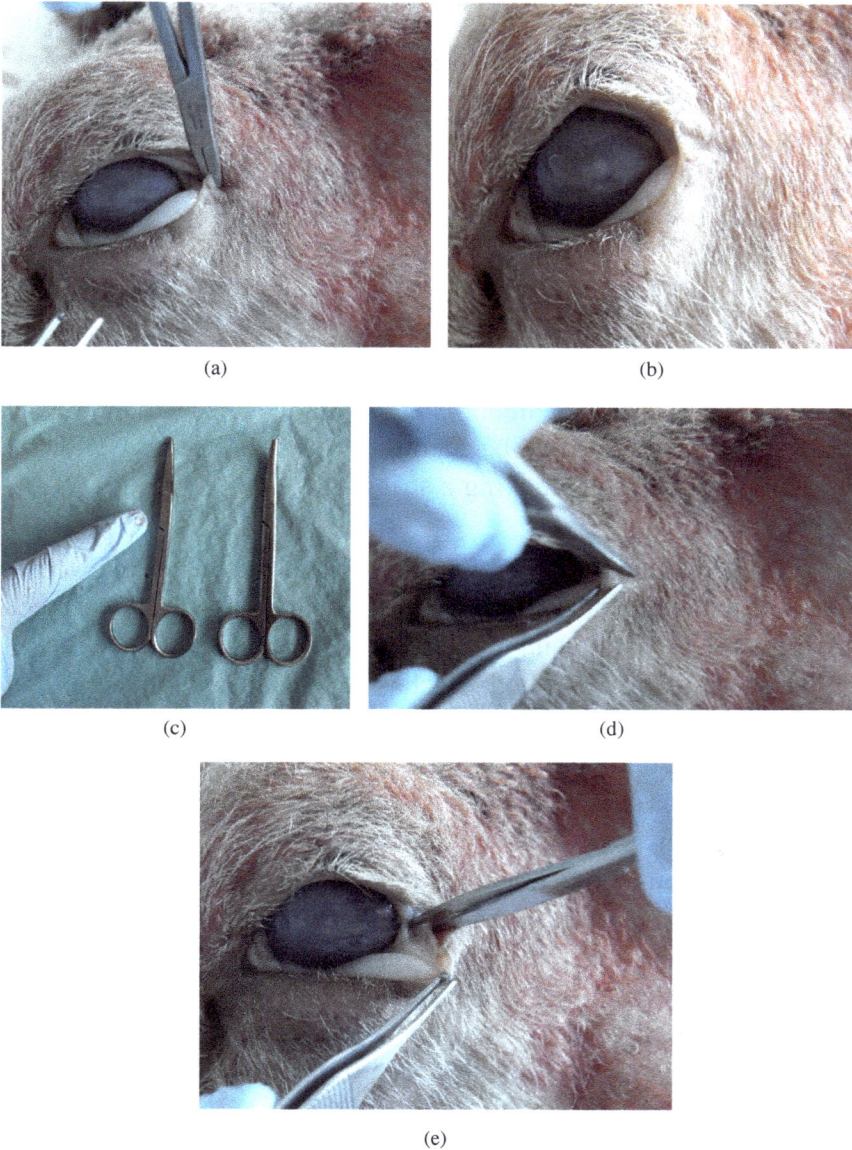

Figure 1.21 (a) and (b) Left lateral palpebral tendon is crushed by applying arterial forceps for one minute; (c) Straight tenotomy scissors are then used to cut the crushed tendon; (d) Pass the tip of the scissors along the lateral canthus to feel for the tendon and cut it at the orbital rim i.e. cantholysis; (e) Lower eyelid should now be free to relieve the intraorbital pressure.

or by a tonometer; however, the measure of intraocular pressure using a tonometer may not be effective in sheep heads.

(b) Local anaesthetic (lignocaine 2% with adrenaline 1:200,000) is injected into the lateral canthus prior to sectioning the palpebral tendon.

(c) The palpebral tendon has been compressed for one minute with artery forceps.

(d) Iris scissors are then used to cut the compressed lateral canthus at the rim of the orbit.

(e) If decompression is not achieved, the inferior crus, a branch of the lateral canthal ligament is cut, which is termed cantholysis. The inferior crus may be identified by strumming it with the scissors similar to plucking a string.

The lateral canthus is multi-structured and contains Lockwood's suspensory ligament. The intraocular pressure was raised by injecting retro-orbital saline and glycerine.

This simulation method teaches a vital technique that can prevent permanent loss of sight, and a cadaver is not generally available for training due to the expense, particularly in a war zone, where the chaos makes everything more difficult. The retrobulbar haemorrhage is simulated by viscous glycerol which is thick enough to be retained behind the globe. It is difficult to measure the release of fluid pressure for which a tonometer may be used. Due to the lack of time and laboratory regulations which required the immediate disposal of the sheep's heads at the end of the course, the trainees were marked using a video recording. This also enabled the course to be taught online from which the trainees could be further assessed.

Eight of the 11 trainees failed the pre-training assessment, but all passed post training (Figure 1.22). Marks were 16/30 pre-training and 26/30 post-training, although seven out of the 11 candidates had previous experience of performing a cantholysis.

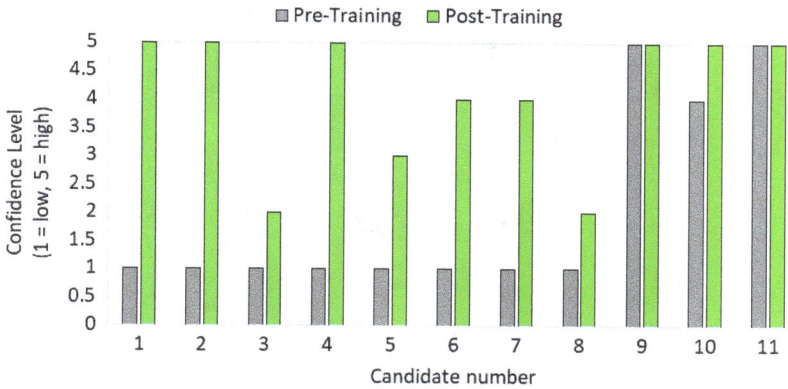

Figure 1.22   Pre- and post-training levels for canthotomy and cantholysis show a substantial post-training improvement in eight out of 11 cases.

All candidates were assessed by an ophthalmic surgeon. Unfortunately, this crucial operation is usually missing from emergency surgery courses.

The Wilcoxon signed-rank test applied to the HTA data showed that canthotomy training elicited a statistically significant increase in participant scores compared to pre-training scores ($Z = -2.431$, $p < 0.05$) with a mean post-training score of 23.27 compared to a pre-training score mean of 16.0. Although scores improved in nine of 11 canthotomy post-training candidates, two trainees were already skilled.

Skill Station 4: External Pin Fixation for Mandibular Fractures

Mandibular fractures are commonly reduced and fixed using intermaxillary Erich arch bar or with dental eyelet wiring loops. Given the equipment options, internal fixation with miniature plates and screws provides improved stability.

An acrylic-filled silicone tube can be used for the fixation of a fractured mandible. Figure 1.24 shows an ingenious external pin fixation consisting of a combination of self-tapping orthopaedic

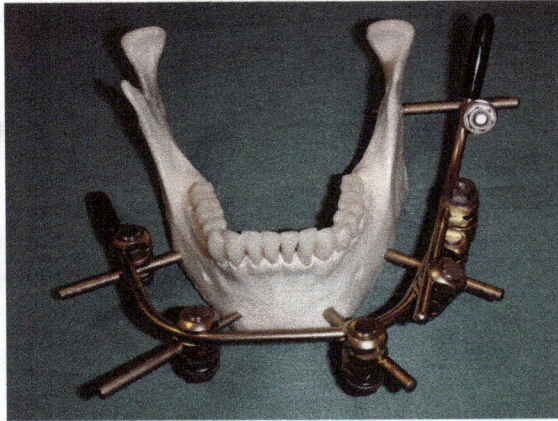

Figure 1.23 This elaborate external pin fixator can stabilise comminuted mandibular fractures but is expensive and needs expert supervision.

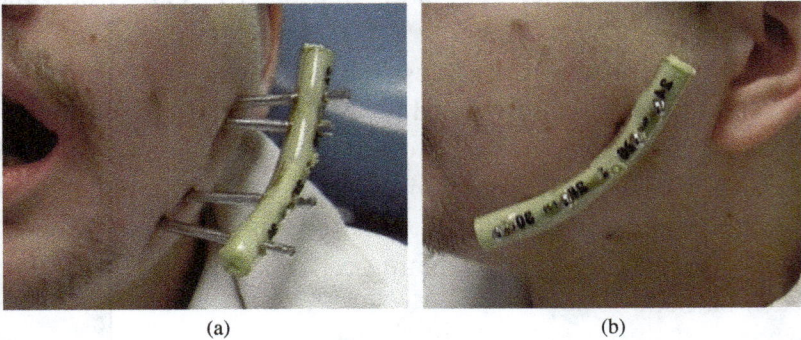

(a)   (b)

Figure 1.24 External pin fixation using self-tapping orthopaedic screws stabilised by an acrylic-filled silicone chest tube. Attribution: Mike Perry.

screws as fixator pins to localise the fracture components. They are stabilised by the acrylic-filled silicone tube instead of a metal connecting bar.

Figures 1.25 and 1.26 show another example of the creative use of available technology in an austere environment. In a Misrata field hospital, Libya (2011), an orthopaedic pin fixation system designed for use with hand fixation is implemented to treat a

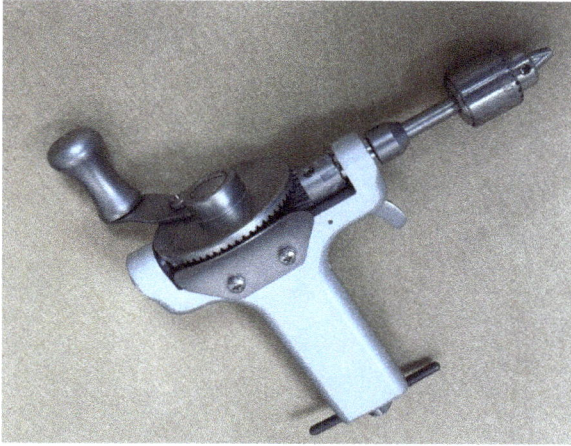

Figure 1.25   Manual orthopaedic drill.

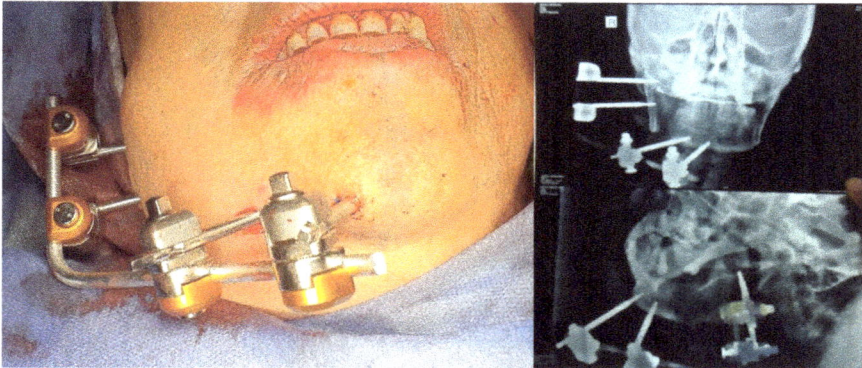

Figure 1.26   Application of orthopaedic fixation system to treat mandibular fracture. A four-pin system, two pins parallel to each other through the right side of the mandible.

mandibular fracture. This allows manipulation and reduction of the fracture after pin placement and guarantees sufficient stiffness of the frame.

Although the sheep's head provides an ideal model for most training, the major drawback is the anatomical difference between

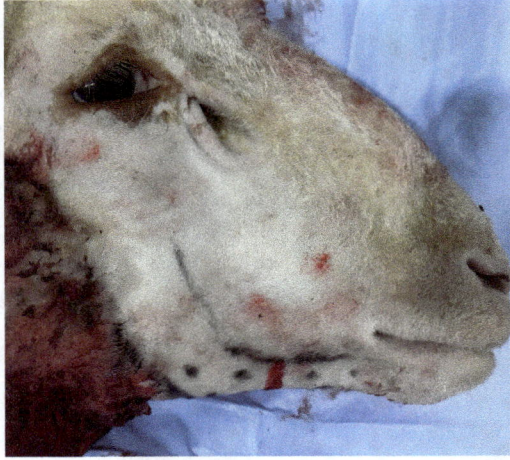

Figure 1.27   Marking the fracture in red and the screw sites in black.

the human dentition and the sheep's dental morphology, which makes intermaxillary fixation difficult (Figure 1.27).

Instruments:
(1) Electric or manual screwdriver with four changeable bits.
(2) Four 7.5 × 80 mm bone screws: Their spiral threads convert torsional forces into compression of the fracture.
(3) Flexible 11-mm diameter silicone tube.
(4) Scalpel number 11 to create skin incisions.
(5) Mosquito forceps to expose the bone.
(6) Acrylic monomer and polymer.

Stab incisions are made on each side of the pre-marked red fracture line and with a curved Dunhill clip or mosquito forceps; the stab wound is stretched to gain access to the bone.

The underlying bone of the stab wound is exposed for the screws using the forceps. The screws are uploaded on the screwdriver of the cordless drill (Figure 1.28).

The first screw is inserted 10 mm from the red fracture line and a further 10 mm to the second screw. The screw is inserted through

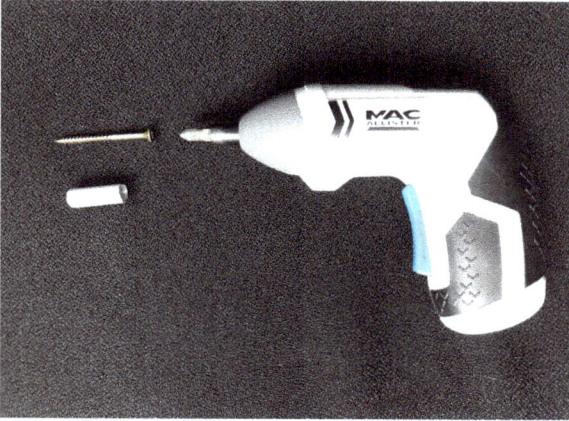

Figure 1.28 Electrical cordless screwdriver.

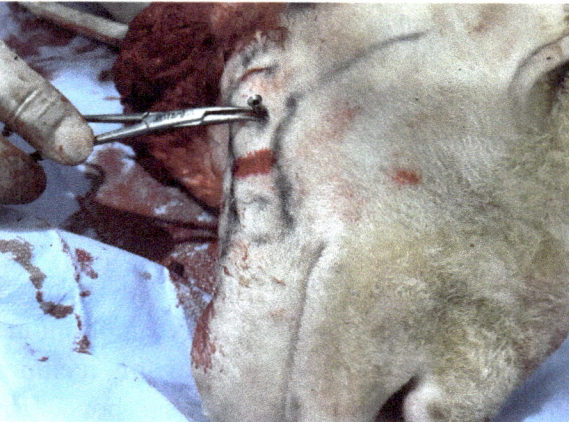

Figure 1.29 Screw is inserted through a sleeve which protects the overlying soft tissue.

a sleeve which protects the overlying soft tissue (Figure 1.29). This is repeated on the other side of the fracture.

The liquid acrylic monomer and the powder polymer are then mixed to achieve a polymerising dough which is then transferred into a split transparent silicone tube to enclose the screw heads and allowed to set.

The screws are then inserted through the silicone tube into the marked screw holes.

They are checked for rigidity, for their parallelism, and that each is at right angles to the surface of the mandible.

The excess material is then trimmed. The polymer sets and gives rigid support for the pins to provide the best possible occlusion and allowed to set (Figure 1.30).

Ten out of 11 trainees failed the pre-training assessment but only one out of 11 failed the post-training test. The mean scores pre- and post-training were 16/40 and 31/40, respectively, indicating improved levels of skill (Figure 1.31).

HTA data when analysed by the Wilcoxon signed-rank test showed that fixation training produced a significant increase in trainee scores compared to pre-training scores ($Z = -2.67, p < 0.01$) with a post-training mean score of 30.8 compared to the pre-training mean score of 15.6. The trainee scores also improved in every one of the eight steps of the fixation (Figure 1.31).

External pin fixation has been performed using specialist metal fixators (Figure 1.23). However, they are difficult to manipulate unlike the acrylic tube and orthopaedic screw model used for this course.

Acrylic and silicone tube are inexpensive, and the silicone mould can be made to any contour which is important in a war zone.

The orthopaedic screws were ideal for this technique, and the shaved sheep's head has appropriate skin and bone. However, anatomically, the dental occlusion is exceedingly difficult to localise whilst fixing the jaws. Despite this, non-specialised trainees showed considerable improvement post training and this model was easy and inexpensive to teach.

Skill Station 5: Erich Arch Bar and Plaster Dental Models

Dento-alveolar fracture management can be simulated on plaster models for the Erich arch bar or dental eyelet loop. The plaster

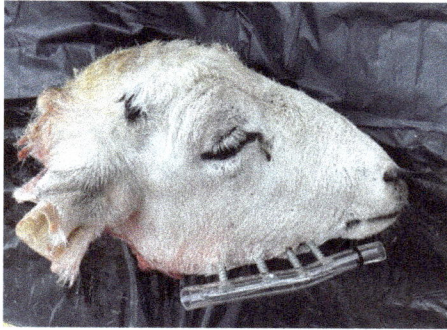

(a)

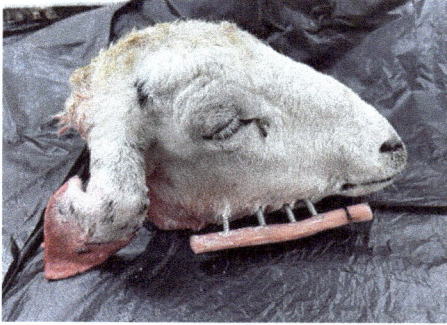

(b)

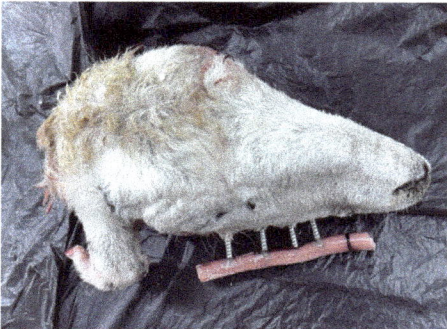

(c)

Figure 1.30 (a) Screws are inserted through the silicone tube into the screw holes; (b) When enclosed by the polymerised acrylic, the silicone tube stabilises the screw heads; (c) A lateral view showing the fixation screws embedded in acrylic.

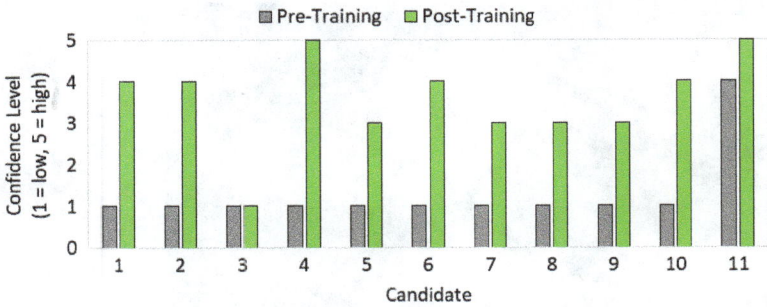

Figure 1.31   Candidate levels pre- and post-training showing the significant increase in the external pin fixation skill.

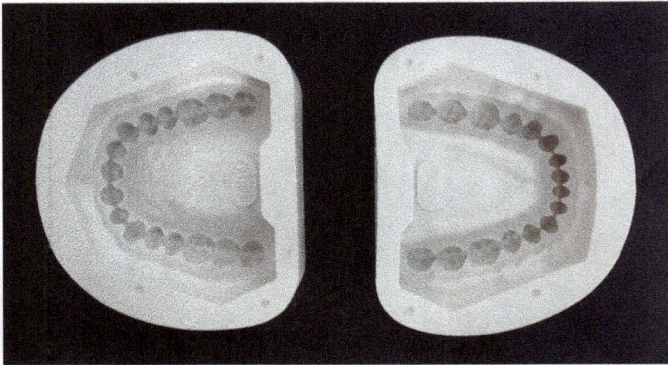

Figure 1.32   Silicone mould used to create the dental plaster models.

model is the most reliable means to teach these skills and is low cost. The Erich arch bar is a simple technique to learn on a plaster model for the non-specialist to manage a fractured mandible (Figures 1.32 and 1.33).

Instruments:
(1) Stainless-steel Erich arch bar adequate in length for two arches.
(2) Stainless-steel wire, gauge 0.5 mm, (SS) 24–26.
(3) Excavator or ligature director to push the wire beneath the cingulum i.e. the neck of the tooth between crown and root.
(4) Scalpel, 15 blade.

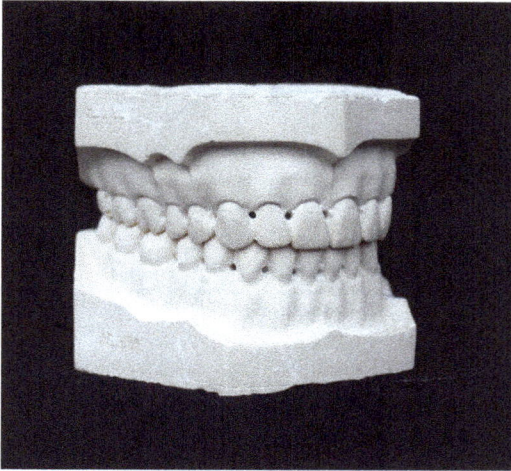

Figure 1.33   Dental plaster models with inter-dental drill holes to facilitate wiring.

(5) Wire-twisting forceps, a wire cutter, a mosquito haemostat, and elastic bands.
(6) The plaster teaching models require a fine, round number-four bur to create an interdental space at the tip of the plaster dental papilla to pass the fixation wires.
(7) Each trainee is provided with six pairs of plaster models and instructions to immobilise a simple body fracture in the lower left premolar region.
(8) A video scenario is also provided to demonstrate IMF fracture management using the Erich arch bar or dental wire loop.

The models were assessed by four oral surgeons.

In clinical practice, the patient's dentition must be checked for gaps, dental occlusion, and periodontal stability to support the Erich arch bar.

The required arch bar length is measured with a wire between the distal surfaces of the last molar teeth on the model; note that the lower arch bar is shorter than the upper (Figure 1.34).

To attach the arch bar to the dentition, pass the first ligating wire through the interdental drill hole from buccal to palatal and then return it buccally through the adjacent mesial gap.

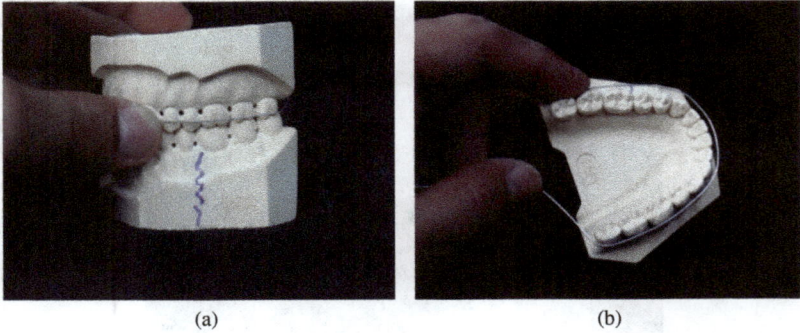

Figure 1.34   Use a length of stainless-steel wire around the model to measure the required circumference of the arch bar.

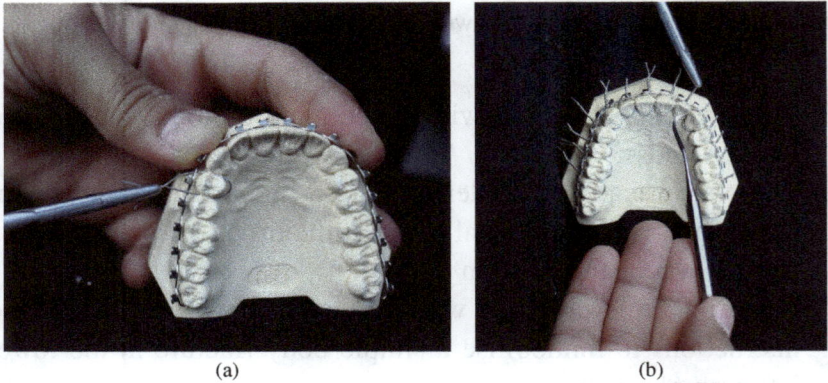

(a)   (b)

Figure 1.35   Twisting the retaining wire loop to lock the arch bar into position.

Use the wire holder to grasp both the ends of the wire and twist twice. Leave a gap initially to insert the arch bar (Figure 1.35).

Repeat this ligating process to pairs of teeth around the dental arch.

Continue to add retaining wires around each tooth through 'interdental' gaps in the plaster model. The wires are returned buccally through the adjacent gap; note that the retaining loop is passed initially underneath the arch bar and returned buccally over it.

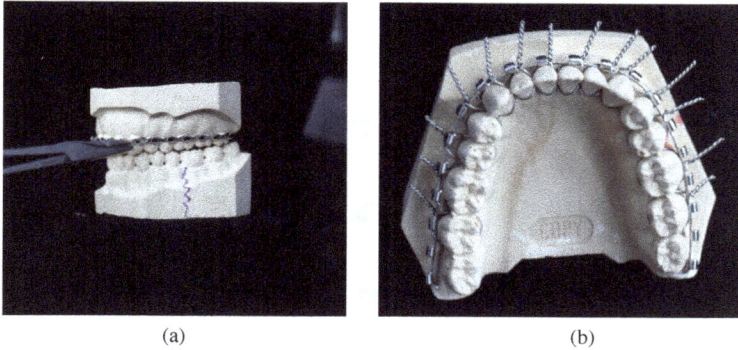

(a)   (b)

Figure 1.36 Excess wire is held with the haemostat when cut so that it does not spring into the eye.

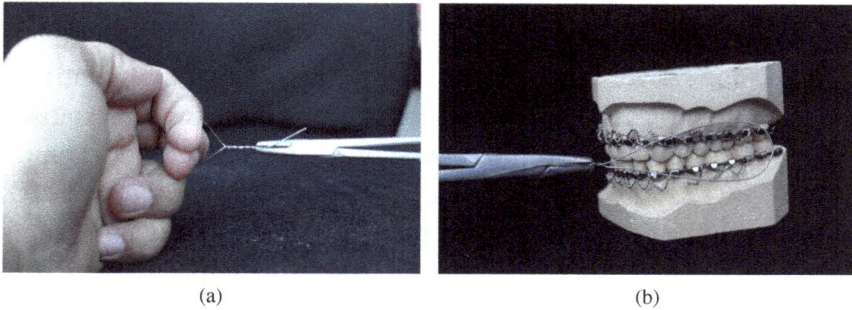

(a)   (b)

Figure 1.37 (a) Intermaxillary fixation is achieved with fish-shape wire loops; (b) Place the IMF wire loops around opposing cleats and use a haemostat to twist them securely.

Always ensure the arch bar cleats (hooks) point apically (towards the tip of the tooth root) for both upper and lower arches.

The retaining wire must be held beneath the undercut of the cingulum (the neck of the tooth crown) with a probe or ligature director to hold it, while twisting the wire to ensure a firm wiring of the arch bar (Figures 1.36 and 1.37).

Ten out of 11 candidates failed the task before training, which decreased to two out of 10 failures post training. The average HTA scores were 15/40 and 27/40, pre- and post-training, respectively.

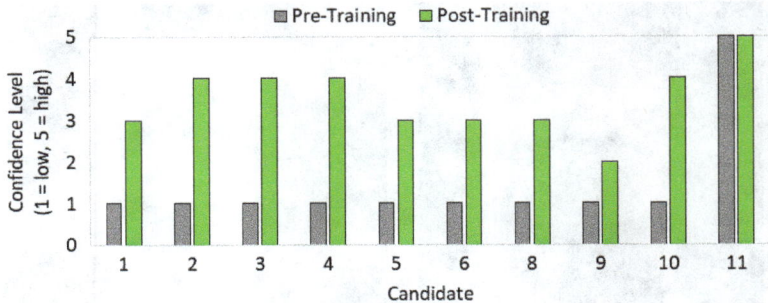

Figure 1.38   Skill levels pre- and post-training for the Erich arch bar station.

The Erich arch bar is an essential maxillofacial skill; however, as seen on the bar chart (Figure 1.38), 10 out of 11 trainees failed the pre-training tasks. This showed the lack of arch bar experience. Despite this, the majority passed post training but with a relatively low average score. The Wilcoxon signed-rank test showed a statistically significant increase in trainee scores compared to pre-training scores ($Z = -2.81$, $p < 0.01$) with a mean post-training score of 26.8 compared to a pre-training score mean of 14.8. Participants scores improved significantly in nine of the 11 steps within Erich arch bar training programme.

Important factors that may have affected the performance could be the allocated time of 25 minutes for this task which was not considered adequate. Fatigue was possibly a contributory factor as this was the final session of a day.

Also, a criticism of plaster models was that the upper and lower jaws were not attached to a stable articulator, lacked tissue and the tongue, all of which would affect wiring performance.

Skill Station 6: Intermaxillary Fixation Using Dental Eyelet Wiring

The eyelet wire loop is an invaluable means of non-specialist management of maxillofacial fractures enabling reduction and fixation to re-establish the occlusion (Figure 1.39).

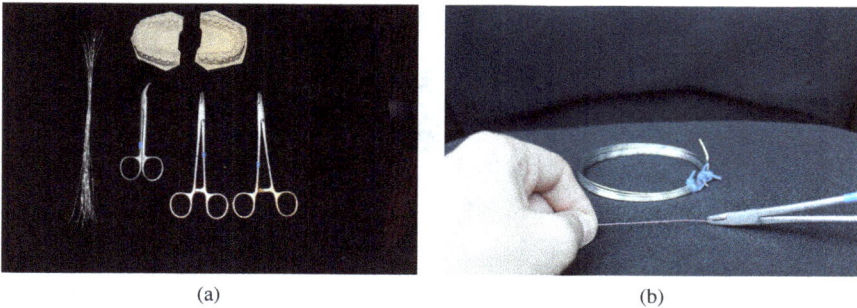

(a)   (b)

Figure 1.39   (a) and (b) Instruments for producing an eyelet wire loop.

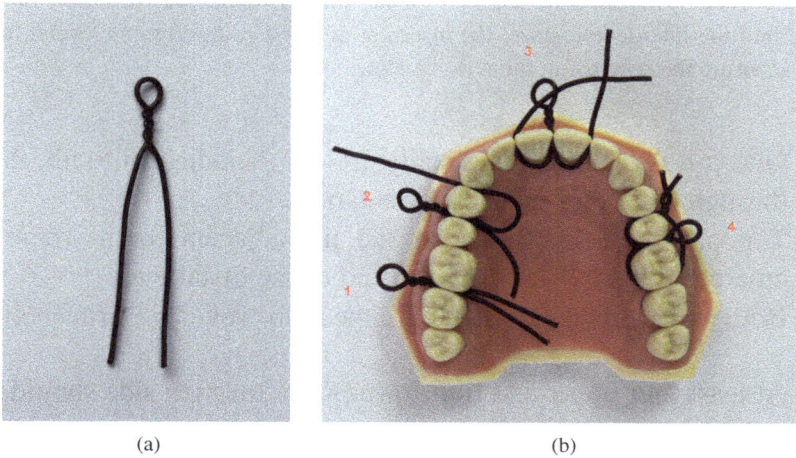

(a)   (b)

Figure 1.40   Note the wire is shown in black for clarity (a) Three-inch wire is folded mid-length and twisted four times to produce the eyelet; (b) Stages of inserting an eyelet wire.

Figure 1.39(b) shows how the wire is fully stretched to three inches before it is bent twice or doubled and twisted. The stainless-steel wire length for each eyelet loop should be 3 in (7.5 cm) after being stretched. Figures 1.40 and 1.41 show the stages of inserting an eyelet wire.

(1) Both free wire ends are then passed palatally or lingually through a buccal interdental space.

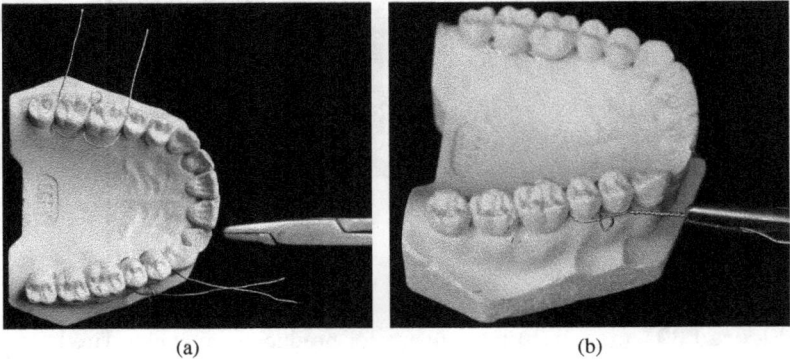

(a)   (b)

Figure 1.41 Process demonstrated on the plaster model: (a) insertion of the wire into the interdental space; (b) insertion of the wire through the eyelet loop and securing the wire using the wire twister.

(2) One end is then passed distally around the adjacent tooth, then through the loop by mesial orientation.
(3) The other end is passed around the adjacent tooth where it emerges to be twisted with the end of the distal wire.
(4) Both wires are then twisted until the loop provides a firm anchor.

At least four upper and four lower loops on each side should be adequate for intermaxillary fixation with firm teeth (Figure 1.42).

On evaluation, only three trainees out of 11 scored a final 30 out of a total of 40 marks. Eyelet loop intermaxillary fixation has similar problems to the Erich arch bar task:

• Fatigue late in the day which may explain a poor pre-training performance.
• Unarticulated stone models require stabilisation when passing wires through the inelastic interdental gaps.
• Plaster model does not take into account missing teeth or irregular occlusion.
• Periodontally mobile dentition excludes dental eyelet loop fixation.

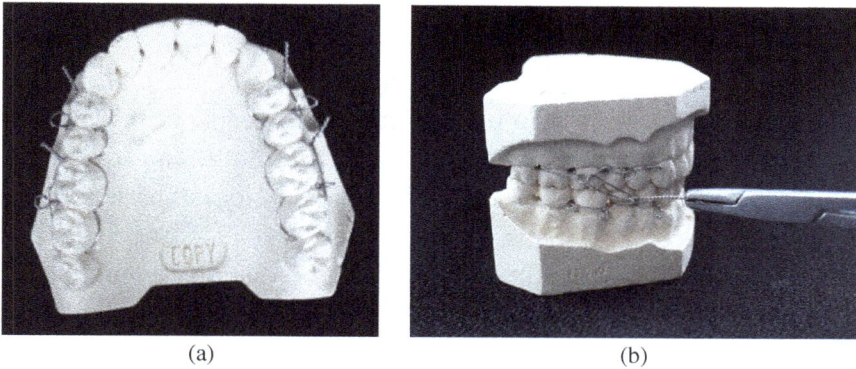

(a)   (b)

Figure 1.42 (a) Four eyelet loops for each side; (b) performing the IMF using the wire twister.

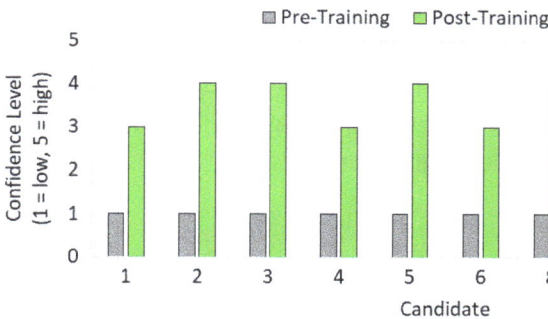

Figure 1.43 Significantly increased ability levels post training for the eyelet wire fabrication and IMF application.

Ten out of 11 trainees failed the pre-training task, whereas all passed the post-training course. The average scores pre- and post-training were 15/40 and 27/40, respectively. The overall ability levels increased significantly in the post-training session.

The Wilcoxon signed-rank test of HTA data showed that eyelet wiring training was statistically significantly improved in trainee scores compared to pre-training scores ($Z = -2.80$, $p < 0.01$) with a mean post-training score of 30.8 compared to a pre-training score mean of 15.55 (Figure 1.43).

Conclusion

The results from our one-day simulated training course show that non-specialist trainees significantly improved their performance in all skill stations following the course curriculum. Improvements were seen in all participants regardless of surgical experience and specialist background. Fatigue contributed to reduced performance in the later skill stations; therefore, the course should be taught over two days at least. Assessment of the skill stations using the HTA developed by specialist surgeons proved to be an adequate and reliable tool to measure the overall performance. As a result, an enlarged programme could be developed to include additional training gaps. One important topic is advanced trauma life support (ATLS) which should ideally be a prerequisite for surgeons in a war zone. Soft-tissue management should also be included as well as the interpretation of head and neck scan images given that 67% of child trauma in war zones is caused by blast injuries.[3–5] Other important areas include psychological trauma and the management of post-traumatic stress disorders.

Appendix — Recommended Videos for the Six Numbered Skill Stations

YouTube links to the procedures covered during the definitive course:

Craniotomy: (1) bit.ly/CNbook1
Prehospital maxillofacial haemorrhage control (nasal balloon): (2) bit.ly/CNbook2
Lateral canthotomy: (3) retrobulbar haemorrhage bit.ly/CNbook3
External pin fixation mandible: (4) bit.ly/CNbook4
IMF with Erich arch bars: (5) bit.ly/CNbook5
How to place eyelet loops: (6) bit.ly/CNbook6

References

1. Holmes S. Primary Orbital Fracture Repair. Atlas Oral Maxillofac Surg Clin North Am. 2021;29(1):51-77. doi:10.1016/j.cxom.2020.11.004.
2. Pringle K, Mackey JM, Modi P, Janeway H, Romero T, Meynard F, Perez H, Herrera R, Bendana M, Labora A, Ruskis J, Foggle J, Partridge R, Levine AC. A short trauma course for physicians in a resource-limited setting: Is low-cost simulation effective? *Injury*. 2015 Sep;46(9):1796–1800. doi: 10.1016/j.injury.2015.05.021. Epub 2015 May 18. PMID: 26073743.
3. Zaggut AW, Rahman MM, Ghanem A, Myers S, Harris M. Training non-specialists for craniomaxillofacial trauma in a warzone setting. *J Dent Open Access*. 2020 Sep. doi: 10.31487/j.JDOA.2020.02.06.
4. Giannou C, Balden M, Molde Å. *War Surgery: Working with Limited Resources in Armed Conflict and other Situations of Violence,* Volume 2 (Royal College of Surgeons; 2014), p. 22.
5. Zaggut AW, Rahman MM, Youssef G, Holmes S, Ellamushi H, Shibu M, Ghanem A, Myers S, Harris M. Craniomaxillofacial war injuries in Misrata, Libya. *J Dent Open Access*. 2020 Aug. doi: 10.31487/j.JDOA.2020.02.05.

Chapter 2

Advanced Trauma Life Support

Sabah Kalamchi, Malcolm Harris, John H. Phillips, and Ian Loh

History of Anaesthesia

The development of anaesthesia was crucial to the development of the speciality of oral maxillofacial surgery.

Oral and maxillofacial surgery evolved through the combined initiatives of notable leaders within dental and medical specialities. William Fry and Harold Gillies were pioneers during the First World War, establishing the first hospital in the UK which specialised in the treatment of face and jaw injuries. Their work could not have progressed without the support of leading contemporary anaesthetists Ivan Magill and Edgar Rowbotham, who realised that complicated invasive surgery required endotracheal anaesthesia. Ivan Magill was the first to use endotracheal anaesthesia and suction equipment while performing dental surgery, which transformed dentistry from the precarious anaesthetic face mask to safe extensive procedures with the endotracheal tube. This was developed at Queen Mary's Hospital Sidcup and changed a surgical 'autocracy', where one surgeon performed all the tasks, to a fully integrated process, where the surgeon, anaesthetist, and a radiologist contributed to the whole process of the specialised craniofacial operation (local anaesthesia of the face is covered in detail in Chapter 4).

Introduction

There has historically been a high prevalence of craniofacial trauma in battle due to the exposure of the head and face. However, craniofacial injuries have been reduced by the use of protective helmets and seat belts and by the introduction in 1975 of advanced trauma life support (ATLS) training programmes.[1] These courses teach skilled trauma management and are based on ABCD principles, which are the maintenance of the Airway, Breathing, Circulation, and the management of Disability.

The treatment of craniofacial trauma patients requires particular cooperation and clear communication between a surgeon and anaesthetist, as they have to share the same anatomical structure, in particular the airway.

Such cooperation must include:

- the control of haemorrhage;
- concern for a possible cervical spine injury;
- a fracture of a skull base;
- facial fractures.

Any delay in airway management will lead to an increased morbidity or even mortality in the prehospital or hospital setting.

Airway and Maintenance of Breathing

The primary action with an unconscious patient is to protect and secure the airway with the following manoeuvre:

The head tilt, chin lift, and jaw thrust (Figure 2.1).

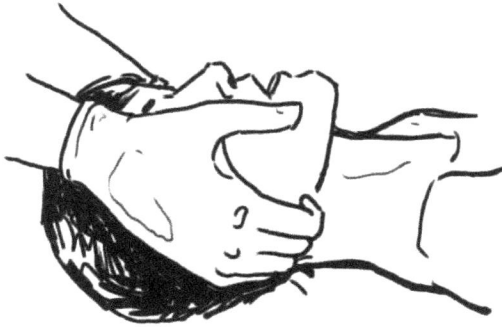

Figure 2.1 Head tilt, chin lift, and jaw thrust.

It is important to position the hands bilaterally to advance and support the mandible without the risk of displacing a cervical spine fracture. Any patient sustaining an injury above the clavicle or a head injury resulting in an unconscious state should be suspected of having a cervical spine injury and should be immobilised and examined with a computed tomography (CT) scan until this is ruled out (Figure 2.2).

The important factors are as follows:

- Establishment of the airway.
- Establishment of whether this is an emergency or an elective surgical procedure.
- Is mask ventilation safe management?
- Is a guided anaesthetic induction to be preferred to conscious intubation?
- Is the laryngoscope view compromised by the surgery?

The induction of anaesthesia can be via:

- inhalation such as nitrous oxide;
- a volatile liquid, such as ether, halothane, or sevoflurane;

- an intravenous route: propofol, thiopentone, etomidate, keta-mine, midazolam, and an opioid agonist, such as fentanyl;
- intramuscular induction agents, such as ketamine, tiletamine and zolazepam, and opioids.

However, craniofacial injuries always complicate mask ventila-tion and pre-oxygenation of the patient. This makes intubation complicated.

High-flow nasal oxygenation can be utilised assuming there is no nasal rhinorrhoea or skull base fracture. If the patent is ade-quately oxygenated, a physical examination to decide the appropri-ate airway technique can be performed.

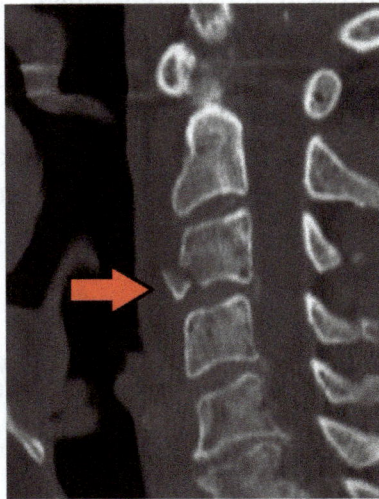

Figure 2.2   Cervical spine teardrop fracture of the C3 vertebra (a sagittal CT scan).

Source: Image licensed under CC BY-SA 4.0. By James Heilman, MD.

Airway Control Techniques

The comparison of airway control techniques can be seen in Table 2.1.

Table 2.1 Comparison of airway control techniques.

Advantages	Disadvantages
Oral endotracheal intubation	
• The quickest technique of securing an airway • Useful in upper and middle third facial fractures	• Cannot be used with maxillo-mandibular fracture fixation
Nasal endotracheal intubation	
• Can be employed in maxillary and mandibulary fractures • Videolaryngoscopy can assist if the cervical spine is compromised • Can be secured to the nasal columella	• Epistaxis • The naso-orbital-ethmoidal (NOE) bone complex is a delicate structure. Damage may result in severe facial dysfunction. The management remains controversial. Surgeons should perform comprehensive clinical examination with radiographic analysis prior to any attempt of Nasal intubation
Conscious flexible fibre optic nasal endotracheal intubation	
• Gives an invaluable view of the airway • Patient is able to maintain oxygenation • Useful in maxillo-mandibular fracture fixation	• Epistaxis • Not used in nasal fractures • Not used in base of skull fractures
Submental intubation	
• Can be employed for both nasal and maxillo-mandibular fracture fixation • Complete occlusion • Operating field is clear	• Invasive • Maximum duration of use is 24–48 h • Risk of infection and salivary fistulae
Tracheostomy	
• Definitive airway • Better pulmonary aspiration • Long-term ventilation possible	• Invasive and fraught with complications • Post tracheostomy care • Risk of tracheal stenosis

Details of Airway Control Techniques

The non-surgical option to establish the airway is a cuffed endotracheal tube (Figure 2.3) which is passed down below the vocal cords (Figures 2.4 and 2.5), but in emergency cases, where long-term ventilation is required, a surgical airway such as a tracheostomy may be necessary.

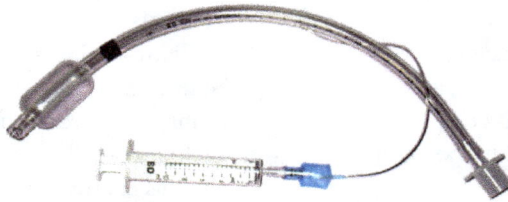

Figure 2.3   Cuffed endotracheal tube.

Source: Image licensed under CC BY-SA 2.5. Sondeintubation.jpg: bigomar2; derivative work: Luigi Chiesa.

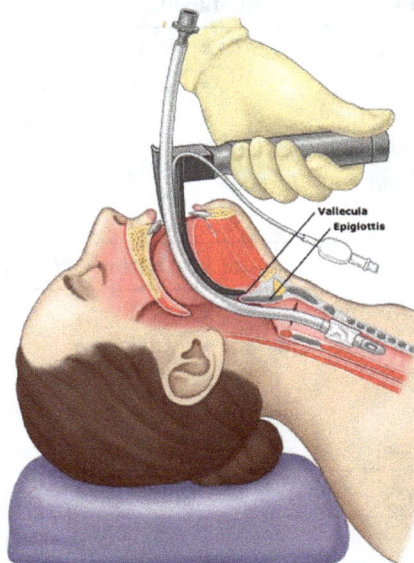

Vallecula
Epiglottis

Figure 2.4   Endotracheal airway being inserted with a laryngoscope.

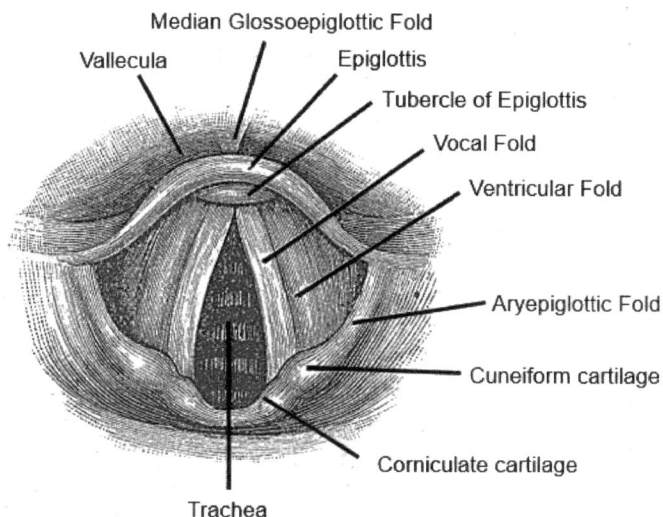

Figure 2.5   Anatomical diagram of the separated vocal cords showing the trachea below (from Gray's Anatomy).

Surgical Airways

Emergency Surgical Cricothyroidotomy

This is an incision made through the skin and cricothyroid membrane between the thyroid and cricoid cartilages (Figure 2.6). It establishes a patent airway to overcome any obstruction, such as an inhaled foreign body, angioedema, or orofacial trauma. The cricothyroidotomy is nearly always performed as a last resort in cases where orotracheal and nasotracheal intubation is impossible or contraindicated. It is easier and quicker to perform than a tracheostomy, does not require manipulation of the cervical spine, and has fewer complications. However, this technique is only intended to be a temporary measure until a definitive airway can be established.

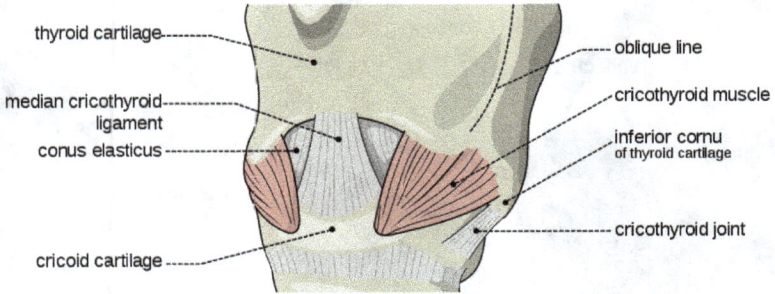

thyroid cartilage

oblique line

cricothyroid muscle

median cricothyroid
ligament

conus elasticus

inferior cornu
of thyroid cartilage

cricothyroid joint

cricoid cartilage

Figure 2.6   Cricothyroidotomy incision site.

Source: Image licensed under CC BY-SA 2.5. By Olek Remesz. wiki-pl: Orem, commons: Orem. Own work based on: Gray951.png.

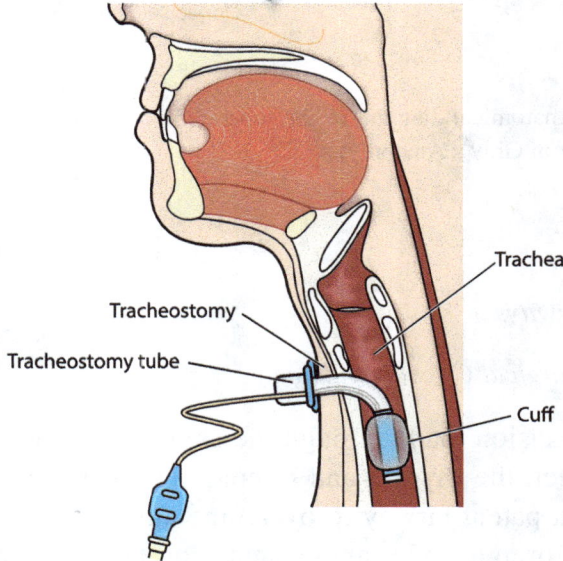

Trachea

Tracheostomy

Tracheostomy tube

Cuff

Figure 2.7   Tracheostomy tube *in situ*.

Tracheostomy

Tracheostomy (Figure 2.7) requires a neck incision to create a direct airway into the trachea through a tracheostomy tube. This allows breathing without the use of the nose or mouth and prevents aspiration into the airway.

First, the anterior neck is prepared and draped for surgery (Figure 2.8). A double towel is placed below the patient's shoulder blades after confirming with a CT scan that the cervical spine is not fractured.

Figure 2.9 shows the anatomical landmarks for the tracheostomy. From left to right are the cricoid cartilage, incision line, and sternal notch.

An incision is made approximately 2 cm above the sternal notch. Bleeding should be arrested with electrocautery. The dissection is extended horizontally into the pretracheal fascia, exposing the strap muscles of the anterior neck (Figure 2.10).

The incision is enlarged with the help of tracheal spreaders and a 3/0 silk suture placed through the inferior aspect of the tracheal incision, which opens the trachea to facilitate the insertion of the tracheostomy tube (Figure 2.11).

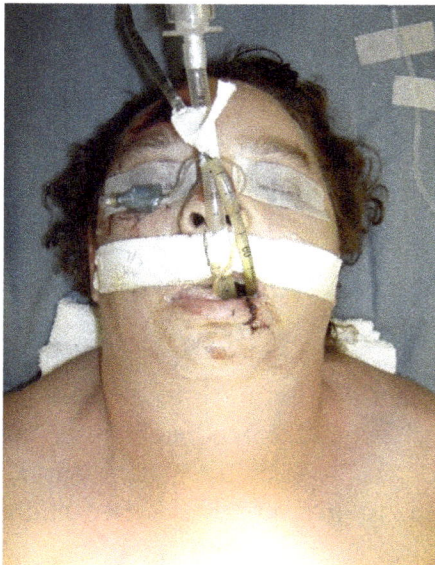

Figure 2.8   Anterior neck prepared and draped for surgery.

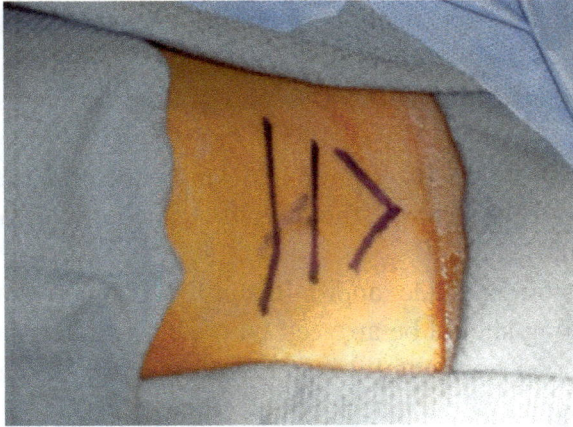

Figure 2.9   Anatomical landmarks for the tracheostomy.

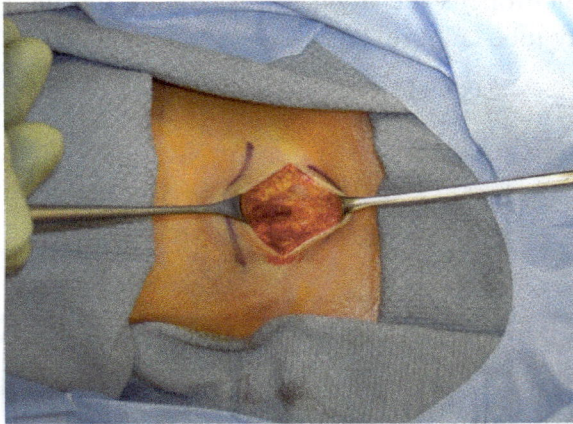

Figure 2.10   Dissection is extended horizontally, and incision is then made through the trachea between the second and third tracheal rings.

The anaesthetist will then retrieve the endotracheal tube from above the incision line and immediately insert a Shiley tracheostomy tube (Figure 2.12) to keep the patient ventilated.

Once the tracheostomy tube is inserted and connected to the ventilator, the CO_2 return is confirmed, and then the original endotracheal tube can be removed.

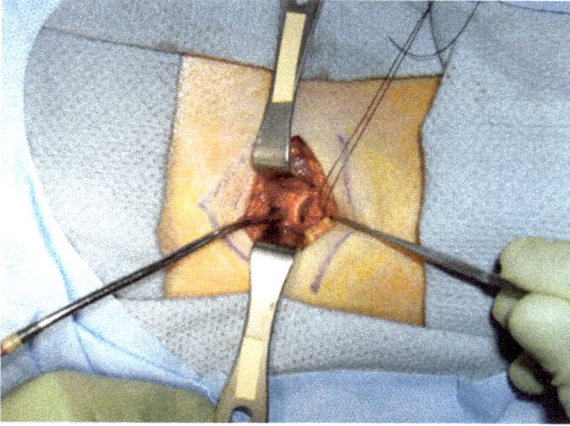

Figure 2.11　Tracheal spreaders and tracheostomy incision.

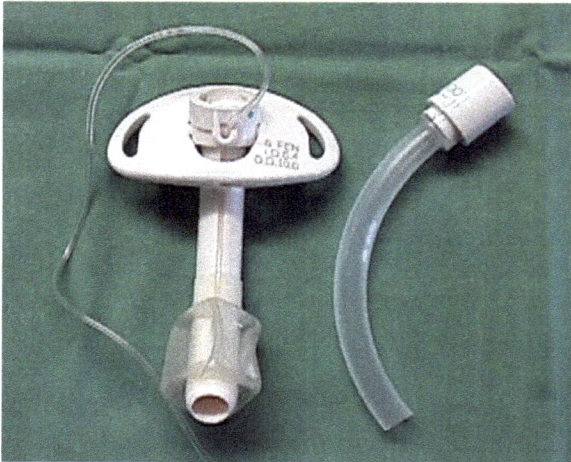

Figure 2.12　Cuffed Shiley tracheostomy tube ready for insertion.

Immediate airway establishment is essential, especially with impaired consciousness and efficient suction of blood and saliva is also essential.

The tracheostomy tube is connected to the yellow ventilator tube and the tracheostomy balloon is inflated (Figure 2.13).

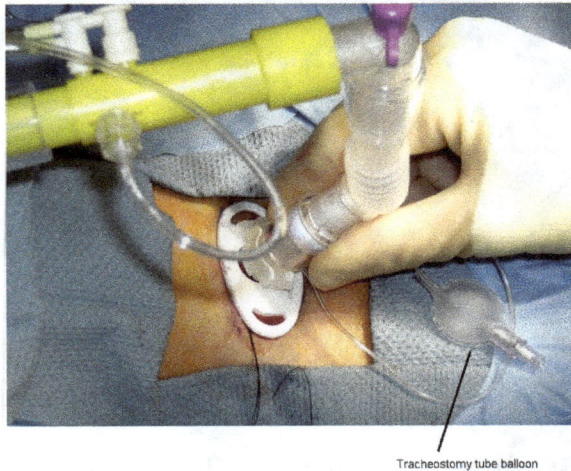

Tracheostomy tube balloon

Figure 2.13   Tracheostomy tube connected to the ventilator tube.

Bone fragments and mobile teeth can now be removed from the mouth, lacerations sutured, and any displaced jaw fractures identified and reduced for fixation.

Important Anaesthetic Challenges

The majority of craniofacial injury patients are kept anaesthetised. In these situations, the surgeon must assist the anaesthetist in decision making:

- Care should be taken with upper third facial fractures which involve the frontal bones, the sinuses and orbit injuries with cerebrospinal fluid (CSF) leaks, especially if nasal intubation, naso-gastric tube and temperature probes are required.
- Middle third Le Fort facial fractures have mobile maxillary components (see Chapter 7 for details on Le Fort).
- Base of skull fractures may present with:
    - epistaxis which obscures the airway;

- facial oedema;
- a CSF leak.
- Posterior displacement of the maxilla can contribute to airway collapse.
- Mandibular fractures may present with trismus, pain, and mal-occlusion.
- The ring-shaped structure of the mandible predisposes to multiple fractures which can obstruct the airway.
- The tongue can be oedematous and posteriorly displaced.
- Loose teeth may be aspirated into the airway.
- Pain-related trismus limits mouth opening.
- Patients with hoarseness or stridor may have laryngeal trauma, especially with burns.
- Trauma-induced vocal cord oedema, arytenoid dislocation, and/or cricothyroid joint disruption may occur.
- Fractures which require intermaxillary fixation (IMF) need intensive care.
- Oedema should be prevented with preoperative corticosteroids.
- The mouth and nasopharynx require suction of blood clot when the throat pack is removed.
- Wire cutters should be available by the bedside in case IMF wires have to be removed.

Circulation

The Management of Surgical Shock

Surgical shock is caused by loss of blood which needs replacement, requiring the insertion of a central catheter line in a vein by an experienced clinician. This enables the transfusion of whole blood or plasma to maintain the blood pressure (Figure 2.14). The insertion of a central venous catheter is well described in this video: https://youtu.be/cmK3hjJYCKA.

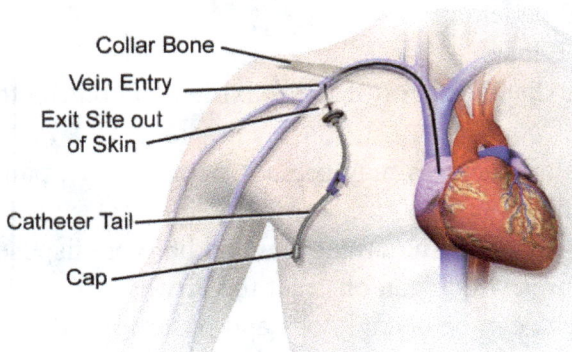

Figure 2.14   Insertion of a central venous line for fluid management.

Arrest of Haemorrhage: Haemostatis

- Exclude any history of hypertension or any medication with anticoagulant action, such as aspirin.
- Antifibrinolytic medication is valuable to arrest bleeding by preventing blood clots from breaking down and is also invaluable for systemic haemorrhage. These agents include aprotinin (Trasylol), tranexamic acid (TXA), epsilon-aminocaproic acid, or aminomethylbenzoic acid. Each is given slowly intravenously.

Table 2.2 shows the control of orofacial haemorrhage.

Facial Laceration Haemorrhage

Bleeding from facial lacerations is a major threat and can be managed by either:

- applying pressure with a gauze pack for 5–10 min, which enables blood clot formation;
- using electrocautery if available;
- clipping and tying off the blood vessel; if the vessel is larger than 2–4 mm, a stick suture can be used (Figure 2.15).

Table 2.2 Control of orofacial haemorrhage.

Site of Injury	Management of the Haemorrhage
Scalp haemorrhage	Identify the bleeding vessels and apply pressure, cauterise, ligate, or over-stitch with a large suture
Oral & facial laceration haemorrhage	Apply direct pressure on bleeding vessels — cauterise or clip and ligate
	Arrest with a tacking suture which is a quick temporary suture intended to be removed
Nasal haemorrhage (epistaxis)	Obstruct the anterior nares with a petroleum jelly gauze pack and/or insert an inflated urinary catheter to obstruct posterior nasal bleeding
Facial burns	Establish airway either with nasal or oral intubation or by tracheostomy and look for signs of inhalation burn injury

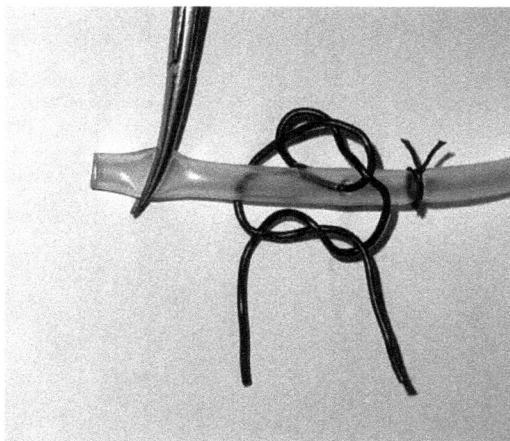

Figure 2.15 Stick suture applied to a large clipped vessel to arrest severe haemorrhage.

Epistaxis (Nasal Haemorrhage)

The nose has an anterior septal confluence of five arteries named Little's area (Figure 2.16), which is prone to bleeding, especially in children. Posterior epistaxis arises from the branches of the spheno-palatine artery in the posterior nasal cavity.

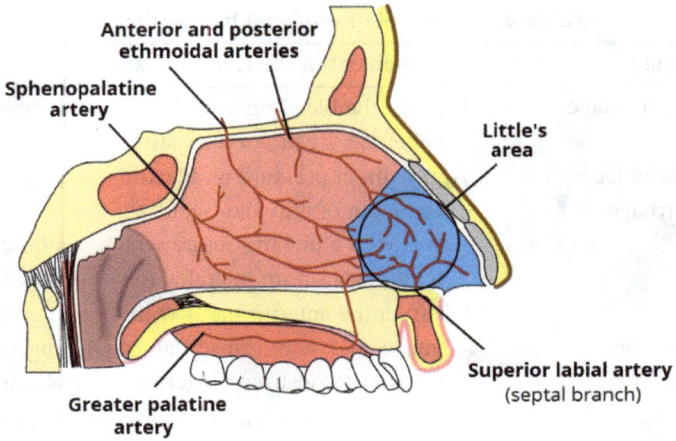

Figure 2.16 Midline diagram of the nasal interior.

Source: Image licensed under CC BY-SA 3.0. Adapted from work by FirstAdmiral via Wikimedia Commons.

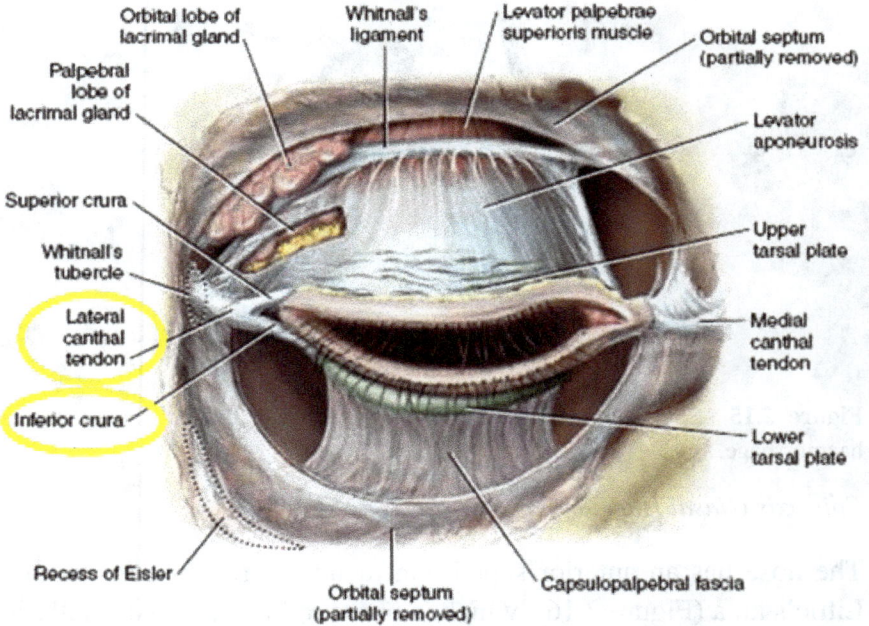

Figure 2.17 Lateral and medial canthal tendons (ligaments) attached to the tarsal plates of the eyelids.

Apart from facial trauma, other causes of epistaxis are picking or blowing one's nose too hard, a combination of trauma and a medication with anticoagulant properties such as aspirin, hypertension, and platelet deficiency (see also the epistaxis section in Chapter 1, Skill Station 2).

Management:

- Always exclude underlying medical and traumatic causes.
- Apply cautery, if available, to stop a bleeding point.
- Insert gauze with a topical vasoconstrictor, such as 2.0% lignocaine with 1/1000 adrenaline, and apply pressure for 5–20 min.
- Nasal bleeding can then be controlled by anterior packing with petroleum jelly gauze or an inflated Foley catheter balloon or both.
- The Foley catheter is inserted through the external nares and inflated with 10 ml of sterile water. It is positioned at the back of the nose so that the inflated balloon tamponades the nasopharynx and secures the catheter in place.
- The balloon is held in place with an umbilical clamp at the anterior nares and a soft dressing is applied to avoid pressure necrosis and protect the columella and septum.
- Pack the anterior nose with layers of petroleum jelly ribbon gauze.
- Antifibrinolytic medication can reduce bleeding by maintaining coagulation.

Retrobulbar Haemorrhage and the Orbital Compartment Syndrome

Management of this is important but the least recognised of ATLS teaching and training skills, although a patient's sight is at risk within minutes of suffering orbital trauma.

Orbital trauma can cause haemorrhage within the bony orbit posterior to the orbital septum. This is a membranous anterior boundary of the orbit that extends from the orbital rim to the eyelids. Haemorrhage behind this partition can produce the *orbital compartment syndrome* by compressing the central retinal artery and adjacent vessels creating ischaemia of the optic nerve and retina with permanent loss of vision. Immediate decompression is necessary.

The medial and lateral canthal tendons hold the eyelids firmly in place (Figure 2.17). Lateral canthotomy is an incision through the lateral canthal ligament to relieve retrobulbar pressure and prevent blindness. If severing the lateral canthal tendon alone does not release the globe, its inferior crura (branch) is also severed. This inferior cantholysis is termed disinsertion.

Treatment must be initiated rapidly to prevent the orbital compartment syndrome. Unfortunately, ophthalmic specialists are not always available in a remote environment and so non-specialists must acquire this sight-saving skill.

The clinical features of the orbital compartment syndrome are:

- intense orbital pain,
- ophthalmoplegia — paralysis or weakness of one or more of the six extra-ocular muscles that control eye movement,
- proptosis,
- reduction of visual acuity with afferent pupillary reflex defect.

The procedure instruments are:

- sterile gauze, gloves, and drapes;
- a 10-ml syringe with a 22–24G needle;
- local anaesthetic (lignocaine 2% with adrenaline 1:200,000) for infiltration into the lateral canthus at the orbital rim to enable the cantholysis incision;
- fine-toothed forceps, needle holder or haemostat, and iris scissors;
- straight arterial forceps and tenotomy scissors;
- ophthalmic antibiotic ointment, such as erythromycin 0.5% or bacitracin (see also Chapter 1 Skill station 3: Lateral canthotomy and inferior cantholysis).

Conclusion

The ATLS programme is essential for any surgeon regardless of the environment and surroundings. The fundamental action for any emergency surgeon is to preserve life, and ATLS provides the training for this. There are other features relevant to ATLS, which can be found in other chapters of this book:

- Radiographs of the dentition, facial skeleton, and cervical spine (see Chapter 9).
- Photographs of craniofacial patients prior to and after injury which are invaluable for facial reconstruction.
- Examination of the cranial nerves.
- Assessment of the patient's mental status.
- Glasgow coma scale.
- Immunisation history for COVID-19, tetanus, or rabies prophylaxis.

In this book, we intend to discuss further craniofacial surgical techniques beyond the ATLS that will significantly improve the quality of life for patients. These techniques are particularly useful for patients in war zones who are unlikely to have access to specialists.

References

1. ATLS Subcommittee, American College of Surgeons' Committee on Trauma, International ATLS working group. Advanced trauma life support (ATLS®): The ninth edition. *J Trauma Acute Care Surg.* 2013 May;74(5): 1363–1366. doi: 10.1097/TA.0b013e31828b82f5. PMID: 23609291.

https://doi.org/10.1142/9781800610194_0003

Chapter 3

Orofacial Pain

Malcolm Harris

Introduction

Pain is a distressing experience associated with actual or potential tissue damage with sensory, emotional, and social components. This is the important and useful biopsychosocial perspective of pain as conceived by Melzak and Wall and later by Engel.[1,2]

Orofacial pain is a wide spectrum of unpleasant experiences which can arise as a consequence of physical or psychological processes or a mixture of both. For this reason, the clinician must have an open-minded approach to its diagnosis. As will be seen, facial pain arising from psychological trauma will be aggravated by surgical intervention, so it is of crucial importance that the clinician does not make the problem worse by embarking on the wrong treatment.

This chapter starts with a discussion of idiopathic orofacial pain and continues with some examples of the varied range of other orofacial pain disorders that it can be mistaken for.

Idiopathic Dental or Facial Pain

The diagnostic obscurity of this pain makes it the most important subject of the chapter. Atypical odontalgia is an idiopathic pain in one or more teeth which has the features of common toothache without any reliable evidence of dental inflammation. It has many names, such as myofascial pain, neuropathic toothache, neurovascular toothache, psychogenic toothache, psychosocial pain, idiopathic toothache, temporomandibular joint pain, hence the simplicity of idiopathic dental pain or idiopathic facial pain are appropriate.

George Engel advanced the biopsychosocial model of Melzack and Wall, which recognises the complex aetiology of idiopathic pains. Melzack and Wall proposed the gate control theory that suggests that the spinal cord contains a 'gate' which can either block or allow pain signals to the brain. These gates are able to differentiate between small and large nerve fibres. Where there is small fibre activity, inhibitory interneurons are impeded, allowing pain stimulation to travel to the brain by which the person will feel pain. Inhibitory interneurons are stimulated by large fibres resulting in diminished information that is transmitted to the brain; therefore, the person will experience less pain. While there is no physical evidence for the existence of these gates, this theory is helpful for understanding pain perception and emotion. With regards to idiopathic facial pain, Engel's **biopsychosocial** structure can be applied in order to avoid unnecessary and irreversible dental treatment (Figure 3.1).

Engel's three domains when applied to a patient's idiopathic facial pain are:

(1) biological, which identifies the origin of the patient's pain as an inherent biological susceptibility;
(2) psychological, which is an underlying psychological trait, such as anxiety or hypochondriasis;

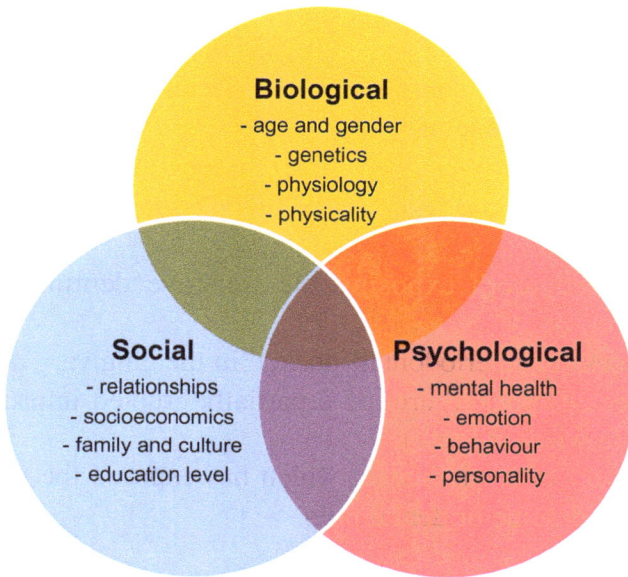

Figure 3.1   Engel's biopsychosocial structure model.

(3) social, which recognises the important role of social or family stress, such as unemployment or homelessness.

This enables the clinician to understand that a persistent or recurrent idiopathic dental pain may not have the inflammatory causes of an infective toothache or the trigger zone of a trigeminal neuralgia and therefore should not be attributed to an inflammatory or neoplastic disorder.

This 'atypical' dental or facial pain may occur daily and is aggravated by any form of dental treatment.

Treatment:

- Detailed explanation and reassurance by an experienced clinician.
- Total avoidance of surgical intervention.
- Management with a tricyclic antidepressant, such as amitriptyline or a selective serotonin reuptake inhibitor e.g. paroxetine.[3,4]

Toothache

Toothache is the most common oral and facial pain. It arises from a variety of dental problems, such as:

- an inflamed dental pulp, usually from an infected or carious tooth;
- a fractured tooth exposing the sensitive dentine or dental pulp;
- an abscess in a periodontal 'pocket' in the gingiva;
- an infected 'pocket' around a partially erupted impacted third molar (a wisdom tooth);
- an erosion of tooth enamel which has exposed the underlying sensitive dentine or dental pulp.

An accurate diagnosis requires a detailed history and examination confirmed by radiographs. The patient usually suffers a throbbing pain aggravated by pressure, chewing, or percussion of the infected teeth, which is aggravated by hot and cold food and drink. Furthermore, the patient may be deceived by pain which appears to arise from the ipsilateral jaw or the maxillary sinus or even from the inner ear. These are 'referred' to as misidentified pains transmitted via connecting trigeminal nerve pathways. A painful dental infection may spread in the face producing tender, palpable submandibular lymph nodes. Relief may be given by drainage of pus, if present, intraorally or surgically extraorally by incision. Less commonly, a severe dental infection may spread as a cellulitis throughout the floor of the mouth into the base of tongue and obstruct breathing and swallowing. This is Ludwig's Angina (Figure 3.2), which impedes the airway by infiltrating the sublingual spaces on both sides of the tongue. The airway must be restored by bilateral sublingual incisions to drain the pus and with oxygen administered through a mask. Antibiotics such as amoxicillin with clavulanic acid are given intravenously or orally eight-hourly.

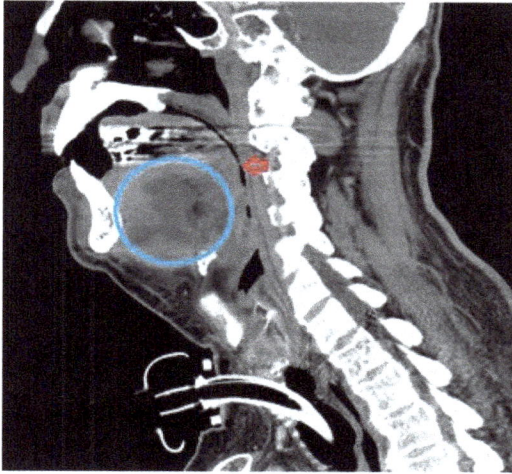

Figure 3.2 Case of Ludwig's Angina: CT scan showing the dense cellulitis expanding the posterior third of the tongue and obstructing the airway (see the red arrow). Attribution: *Southwest Journal of Pulmonary & Critical Care & Sleep* www.swjpcc.com/

Trigeminal Neuralgia

This can be described as a severe 'lightening' pain stimulated by contact with a trigeminal nerve 'trigger site'. Pain lasts from seconds to two minutes, usually involving the lower part of one side of the face. Periods of attacks last from days to months at a time. In severe cases, attacks may happen many times a day. Common analgesics such as paracetamol or ibuprofen do not help with the pain.

Trigeminal neuralgia may be secondary to compression of the trigeminal nerve by a blood vessel, an adjacent tumour, multiple sclerosis or a dental surgical procedure.

It is most common between the ages of 50 and 60. Current management includes control with an anticonvulsant, such as carbamazepine, oxcarbazepine, lamotrigine, or gabapentin or less commonly by neurosurgical relief of the nerve compression.

Herpes zoster is a painful facial rash, commonly known as shingles, and arises as a series of blisters along the distribution of the trigeminal nerve. It is caused by the varicella zoster virus that lies dormant in the trigeminal nerve ganglion following a chickenpox infection and can therefore cause trigeminal neuralgia. Acyclovir, an antiviral drug, taken at 800 mg orally five times daily for 7 to 10 days is the recommended treatment. Alternatively, famciclovir 500 mg orally three times a day can be used.

Glossopharyngeal Neuralgia

This is a similar sharp stabbing pain in the throat and back of the tongue or middle ear. The distribution of the glossopharyngeal nerve is such that the pain can mistakenly diagnosed as having a dental origin. It also responds to anticonvulsants.

Aphthous Stomatitis (Canker Sores)

These are small, painful oral ulcers on the inside of the mouth, the gingivae, buccal mucosa, lips, and tongue. They appear singly or in recurrent groups. In some cases, they may include swollen lymph nodes and pyrexia.

Aphthous stomatitis (Figure 3.3) is not contagious and heals within one to three weeks without treatment. Major aphthous stomatitis may take up to six weeks to heal.

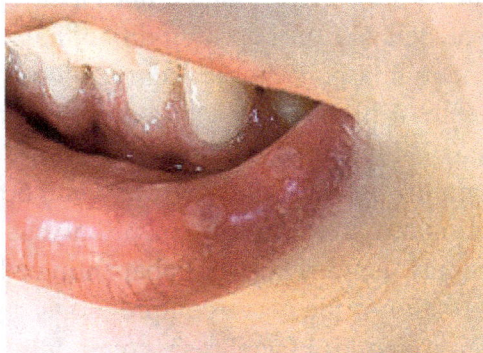

Figure 3.3   Aphthous Stomatitis on lower lip.
Source: Image licensed under CC BY-SA 3.0. By Noorus.

Pain can be managed with benzocaine (Orabase) which acts as a topical anaesthetic and relieves the discomfort.

Recurrent aphthous stomatitis may rarely be a manifestation of the human immunodeficiency virus (HIV) and is treated with antiretroviral (ARV) drugs.

Bell's Palsy: An Idiopathic Facial Nerve Palsy

There is a temporary lack of movement affecting one side of the face which develops within 72 hours and usually recovers within nine months.

An example of the pitfalls of misdiagnosis, despite its neuropathic presentation, Bell's palsy is **not** caused by a fracture of the skull base or surgical damage to the facial nerve. Its origin may be actually linked to the herpes virus, and it is not usually painful. Presentation includes a drooping eyelid or corner of the mouth, eye irritation due to lack of closure, and dribbling of saliva with a loss of taste (Figure 3.4).

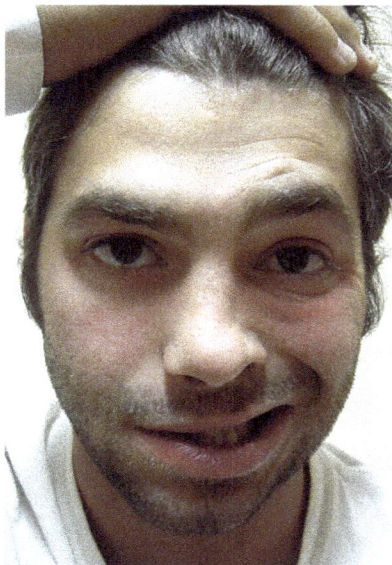

Figure 3.4   VII Nerve palsy.
Source: Image licensed under CC BY-SA 3.0. By James Heilman, MD.

The treatment of Bell's palsy is more effective if started within 72 hours of onset. A 10-day course of prednisolone eye drops and eye ointment is used to stop the affected eye drying out. Surgical tape is required to keep the eye closed during sleep. There is no proof that corticosteroids or antiviral medication are effective.

References

1. Melzack R, Wall PD. Pain mechanisms: A new theory. *Science*. 1965 Nov 19;150(3699):971–979.   doi: 10.1126/science.150.3699.971.   PMID: 5320816.
2. Engel GL. The clinical application of the biopsychosocial model. *Am J Psychiatry*. 1980 May;137(5):535–544. doi: 10.1176/ajp.137.5.535. PMID: 7369396.
3. Rizzatti-Barbosa CM, Nogueira MT, de Andrade ED, Ambrosano GM, de Barbosa JR. Clinical evaluation of amitriptyline for the control of chronic pain caused by temporomandibular joint disorders. *Cranio*. 2003 Jul;21(3):221–225.   doi: 10.1080/08869634.2003.11746254.   PMID: 12889679.
4. Mattia C, Paoletti F, Coluzzi F, Boanelli A. New antidepressants in the treatment of neuropathic pain. A review. *Minerva Anestesiol*. 2002 Mar;68(3):105–114. PMID: 11981519.

Chapter 4

Orofacial Surgery

Abdulhakim Zaggut and Malcolm Harris

Introduction

This chapter covers the management of common facial lesions emphasising the invaluable use of local anaesthesia (general anaesthesia is covered in Chapter 2).

Suturing a facial wound requires a local or general anaesthetic. As facial appearance is important and affects the treatment outcome, it is necessary to pay attention to smaller elements that may be ignored in situations where time is limited. Thanks to advancement in technology, such as smartphones, photographs of a patient (prior to, during, and post) injury have become invaluable for facial morphology assessment and outcome improvement.

Local Anaesthesia of the Face

Facial and oral anatomy is complex, and an understanding of the nerve supply for each region is vital to achieve appropriate delivery of anaesthesia. For example, infiltration or nerve block local anaesthesia (LA) is used when facial laceration suturing is performed.

The maxillary region has thin alveolar bone which makes infiltration anaesthesia effective. Infiltration anaesthesia is a simple procedure and can be administered intra or extra orally. Mandibular bone is thick, and this makes nerve block more effective; however, although uncommon, complications from nerve block can occur, affecting the inferior alveolar nerve such as pain, dysphasia, facial palsy, and trismus.

In the head and neck region, there are 12 motor and sensory cranial nerves. In the craniofacial region, the trigeminal and facial nerves are the most important nerves to anaesthetise (Figure 4.1).

Trigeminal Nerve

The trigeminal nerve is the principal sensory nerve of the mouth and face, and its motor nerve activates the muscles involved in mastication. A small motor and large sensory branches emerge from the side of the pons, near its upper border, and exit the cranial cavity through

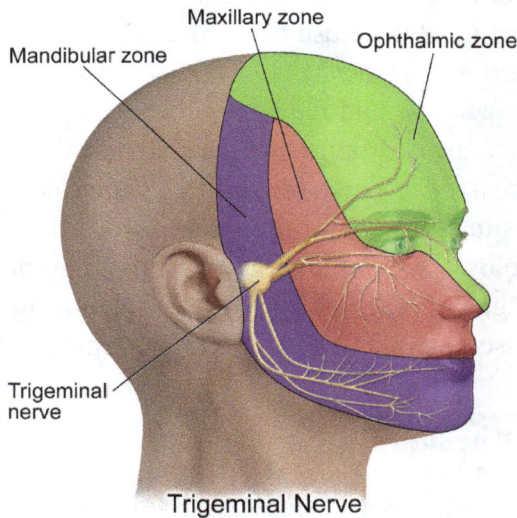

Figure 4.1   Trigeminal nerve sensory branches are the ophthalmic (V1), maxillary (V2), and mandibular (V3).

Source: Image licensed under CC BY-SA 4.0. By BruceBlaus.

the foramen ovale in the base of the skull. The small motor root of the trigeminal nerve passes under the trigeminal ganglion and through the foramen ovale to unite with the sensory root just outside the skull.

Topical anaesthetics can be used to control pain before injecting the local anaesthetic. The local anaesthetic can then be infiltrated around the wound or given as a nerve block. The administration of a local anaesthetic is suitable for short lacerations that can be anaesthetised by injections along the wound margins. Larger lacerations require a nerve block of lignocaine 1–2% with adrenaline (epinephrine) 1:200,000 which takes 5–10 min to be effective, lasting between 45 and 60 min.

Bupivacaine (Marcaine) is a longer-acting anaesthetic agent. The dose is 2–3 mg/kg body weight, and it takes 10–15 min to be effective and lasts 2–4 h. Deep wounds also require a nerve block of the major trigeminal nerve branches (Figure 4.2).

Supraorbital Nerve Block V1

- Insert the needle into the eyebrow at the point where the V1 nerve exits from the skull.

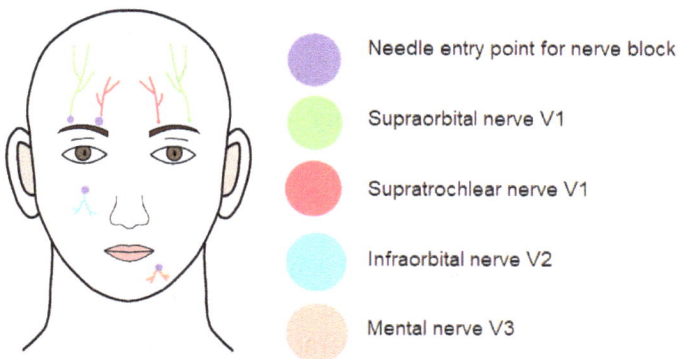

Figure 4.2 Illustration of the entry points for four nerve blocks.

- Inject 1 ml of the anaesthetic solution into the superficial tissues.
- Advance the needle to the bony hard surface.
- Withdraw the needle 1–2 mm away from the bone and inject another 2–3 ml of local anaesthetic.

For a forehead wound above the medial third of the eyebrow, both the supraorbital and supratrochlear nerves need to be blocked on the side of the injury.

Supratrochlear Nerve Block V1

The supratrochlear nerve supplies sensation to the medial upper eyelid, upper nose, and medial forehead. It exits the skull at the medial end of the supraorbital rim, lateral to the area where the rim meets the nose.

- Insert the needle into the soft tissues overlying where the nerve exits the skull.
- Inject 1 ml of anaesthetic solution into the superficial tissues.
- Advance the needle tip downward to the bone.
- Withdraw the needle 1–2 mm away from the bone and inject another 1–2 ml of the solution.
- For a forehead wound above the medial third of the eyebrow, both the supraorbital nerve and supratrochlear nerves need to be blocked on the side of the injury

Infraorbital Nerve Block V2

- The infraorbital nerves supply sensation to the upper lip, cheek, lateral aspect of the nose, and lower eyelid. There is one on either side of the face. The infraorbital nerve comes out of the skull approximately 5 mm below the orbital rim along the vertical line drawn perpendicular to the midpoint of the pupil.

- Insert the needle into the intraoral buccal sulcus at the point where the perpendicular vertical line drawn from the midpoint of the pupil meets a horizontal line drawn from the alar margin of the nose.
- Advance the needle tip 2–3 mm into the tissues.
- Inject 1 ml of solution.
- Advance the needle tip further in a slightly superior direction until it contacts the underlying bone.
- Draw the needle back 1–2 mm and inject another 2–3 ml of the anaesthetic.

Inferior Alveolar Nerve Block V3

With the mouth open wide, the anterior border of the ramus is palpated with the index finger at its greatest concavity. The syringe is positioned diagonally across the mouth, resting on the contralateral premolars. Slowly penetrate the mucosa until bone is contacted. Withdraw slightly and aspirate. If no blood is aspirated, inject 1.5–2 ml local anaesthetic. If blood is aspirated, pull back 5–10 mm and then repeat aspiration prior to injecting 2 ml of local anaesthetic.

This should simultaneously anaesthetise the lingual nerve. The long buccal nerve is anaesthetised separately with 1 ml (Figure 4.3).

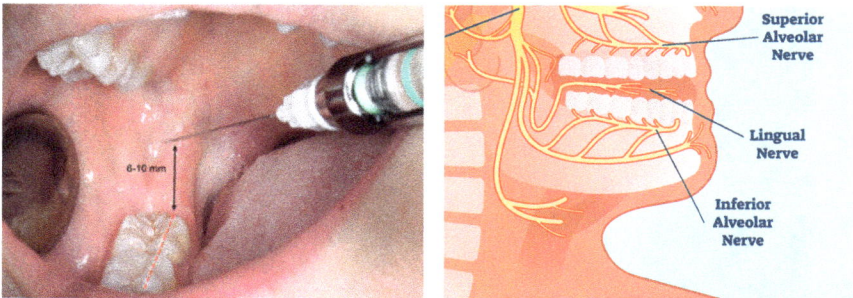

Figure 4.3 Inferior alveolar nerve block deposited medial to the ascending ramus.

Source: Image licensed under CC BY. Copyright © 2014 Medicina Oral S.L.

Mental Nerve Block V3

The mental nerves are the terminal of each mandibular nerve and supply sensation to the lower lip and the skin immediately below it (Figure 4.4). The nerve exits from the mandible 5–10 mm lateral to the apex of the lower canine root.

The mental nerve block is performed in the mouth:

- Insert the needle into the mucosa a few mm below and 5–7 mm lateral to the root of the lower canine tooth.
- Advance the needle tip until it reaches the bone.
- Inject 3 ml of local anaesthetic solution.

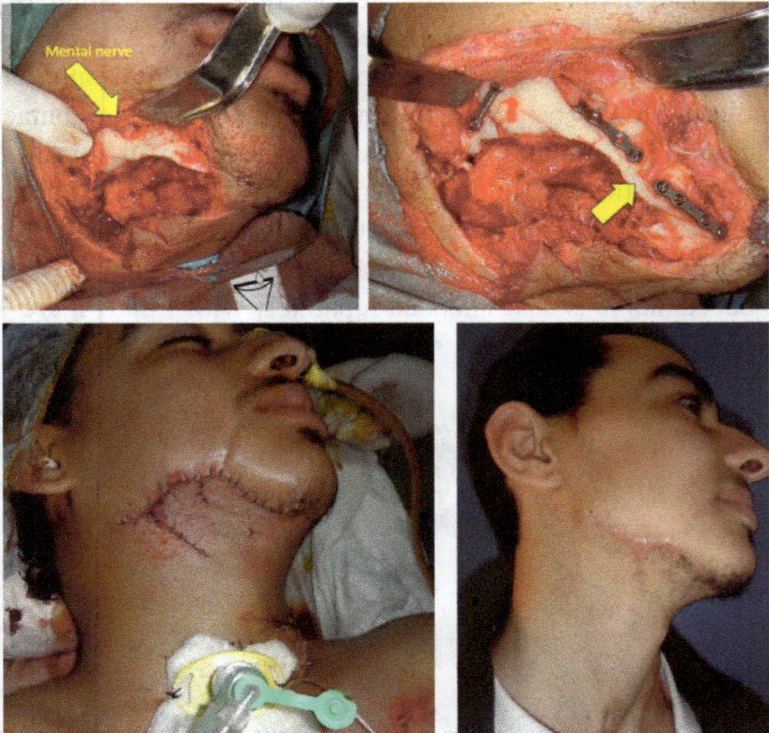

Figure 4.4   War injury with a comminuted mandibular fracture and exposed mental nerve.

Facial Nerve VII

The stylomastoid foramen is an opening through which the facial nerve from the skull passes through into the parotid gland. The nerve in the gland splits into five branches which are the temporal, zygomatic, buccal, marginal mandibular, and cervical branches, as seen in Figure 4.5. It is a mixed sensory and motor nerve.

In addition to supplying the muscles of facial expression, the facial nerve conveys secretomotor fibres to the sublingual and submandibular salivary glands and the lacrimal gland as well as the nasal mucosa. It also carries taste fibres from the anterior two-thirds of the tongue. It is important to be aware of the marginal mandibular nerve that runs deep into the platysma below the mandible; therefore, excision in this area should be made two-fingers width below the mandibular border to avoid damaging the nerve.

The facial nerve also supplies sensory nerve to the tonsils and is part of external auditory meatus.

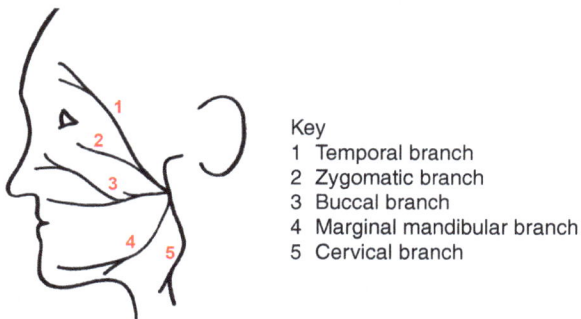

Key
1 Temporal branch
2 Zygomatic branch
3 Buccal branch
4 Marginal mandibular branch
5 Cervical branch

Figure 4.5 Branches of VII cranial nerve (facial nerve) posterior auricular nerve.

Forehead Lacerations

A full-thickness forehead laceration involves skin and the underlying muscle and usually exposes the bone of the skull. Such wounds must be repaired in layers to prevent contour irregularity (Figure 4.6).

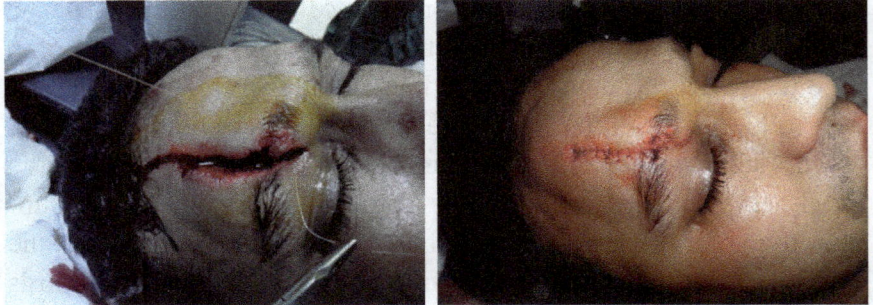

Figure 4.6   Forehead lacerations sustained by blast injury.

Frontal Sinus Fractures

The paired frontal sinuses are at the centre of the forehead, above the bridge of the nose. A computed tomographic (CT) scan of the head is required prior to neurosurgery. If depressed, the anterior sinus wall requires elevation to be immobilised with mini-plates and screws before closing the wound.

Scalp

Full-Thickness Scalp Lacerations

The surrounding hair should be shaved to enable examination of the wound. The muscle and fascia should be brought together with simple or figure-of-eight 3/0 absorbable sutures. The overlying skin is repaired with 5/0 simple sutures (Figure 4.7).

Full-thickness scalp lacerations can cause significant blood loss which is controlled by closing the galea layer. This sheet of connective tissue bridges the gap between the occipital and frontalis muscles forming the middle third of the scalp. Closure of the aponeurosis galea layer also prevents infection from spreading under the entire scalp. Antibiotics help to prevent this serious complication.

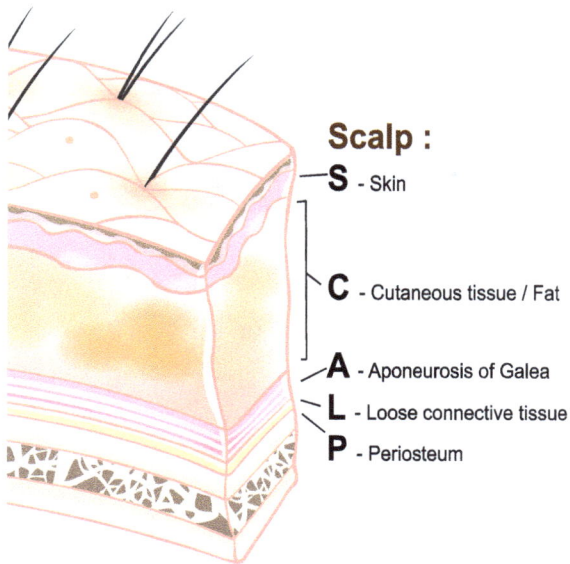

Figure 4.7 Five layers of the scalp.

Facial Lacerations

Auricular trauma

Pain and swelling that occur during the first few days after an ear injury indicate a sub-perichondrial haematoma (Figure 4.8). This auricular deformity is known as 'cauliflower ear' and is a feature of boxers and rugby players. Treatment is to remove the sub-perichondrial blood and prevent its reaccumulation. For this lesion, use 4/0 or 5/0 absorbable interrupted sutures. If the cartilage margin is highly irregular, gently trim the edge under a local anaesthetic to smooth it out, being sure to cleanse the wound of all foreign material. If dirt is embedded in the cartilage, it should be carefully excised to remove the particles.

No sutures need to be placed in the cartilage, but when placing sutures in the skin of the ear, try to include the perichondrium which is the thin layer of loose tissue overlying the cartilage. In this way,

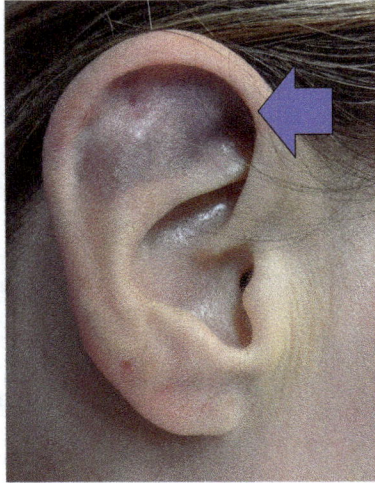

Figure 4.8   Mild auricular haematoma after drainage.
Source: Image licensed under <u>CC BY-SA 4.0</u>. By James Heilman, MD.

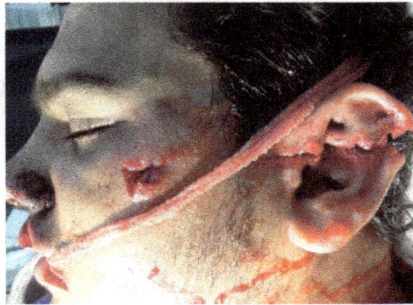

Figure 4.9   Blast injury: exposed severed ear cartilage must be covered with skin.

the cartilage is brought together as the skin is repaired. Here, use 4/0 or 5/0 non-absorbable interrupted sutures (Figure 4.9).

Labial Lacerations

The vermilion border is the red margin of the lips. It is important to realign lacerations of the vermilion border to prevent a notice-

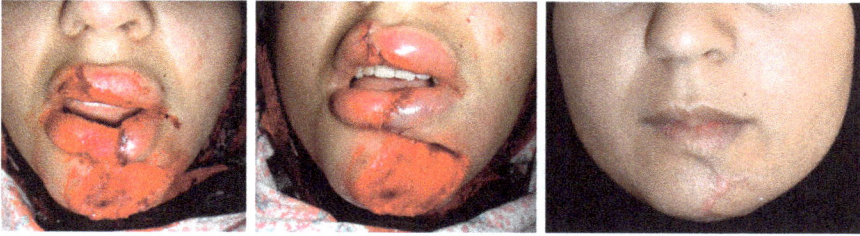

Figure 4.10 Blast injury sustained on lower and upper lips and post-operative photo. Misrata, 2011.

able irregularity (Figure 4.10). The vermillion of the lip is a mucosal surface which can be divided into two parts. The outer part of the lip is the dry mucosa, and the mucosal surface that lies against the teeth is the wet mucosa. It is important to align the border between these two surfaces to prevent irregularity. These borders are best treated by using a nerve block for the repair of lacerations or injecting local anaesthetic a few millimetres away from the wound edge, waiting 5–10 min for the swelling to resolve.

Partial-Thickness Lacerations that Cross the Vermillion Border

- The key to a successful repair is to approximate the vermilion border as well as possible by aligning the red/white margin first. Place the initial suture just above the vermilion border in the white lip skin using a 5/0 or 6/0 suture.
- If the stitch is not well placed, remove it and repeat.
- Place the remaining sutures in the lip skin (5/0 or 6/0) and lip mucosa (4/0 or 5/0).

Full-Thickness Lacerations

- With full-thickness lip lacerations, the outer skin, labial muscle, and mucosa have separated. Such full-thickness lip lacerations can be repaired in layers. Satisfactory primary repair is possible even if one quarter of the upper or lower lip is lost. Whilst suturing, it helps to place a gauze swab intraorally between the lip and gingiva to prevent any bleeding.

- If bleeding is significant, inject with lignocaine 1% with adrenaline 1:200,000 to control bleeding. However, if the bleeding is coming from a cut artery clip and suture with a 4/0 absorbable suture.
- Repair the inner aspect of the lip first using an absorbable 4/0 suture and try to evert the edges.
- To repair the muscle, use 3/0 or 4/0 absorbable sutures. The first suture of this repair should align the margins of the vermillion–cutaneous border, placing one or two sutures in the muscle layer initially.
- Careful inspection of the wound surface will reveal that the muscle and mucosa have different appearances and textures. Take care not to catch any mucosa in the deeper stitches to avoid distortion.
- Irrigate the wound with warm water or saline after the mucosa is closed.
- Tie four knots in lip sutures as they often come undone.

Intraoral Mucosal Lacerations

- Infiltrate 1% lignocaine with 1/200,000 adrenaline.
- Avoid intraoral damage as the tissue is delicate.
- Avoid the parotid duct which opens opposite the mesial buccal cusp of the upper second molar.
- Insert small bites and evert the edges with 4/0 sutures.
- When repairing the oral mucosa, carefully close the lesion using a 5/0 suture. First, suture the subcutaneous layer, then suture the overlying skin.
- Avoid branches of the facial nerve.

Tongue Laceration

(See Chapter 12 for examples and pictures)

A tongue laceration can be painful and tend to bleed and become swollen. The wound prevents speech, eating, and swallowing and may obstruct the airway. The control of the pain, haemorrhage, and the airway are of primary importance.

Management

Apply a gauze swab with firm pressure to stop the bleeding. If bleeding does not stop, a significant laceration must be sutured.

If the vessel is larger than 2–4 mm, haemostasis can be achieved by tying the end of the vessel using a stick suture (Figure 4.11).

Intravenous antifibrinolytic medication, such as tranexamic acid (TXA), will also promote clotting.

A major lingual laceration may require a tracheostomy (Figure 4.12).

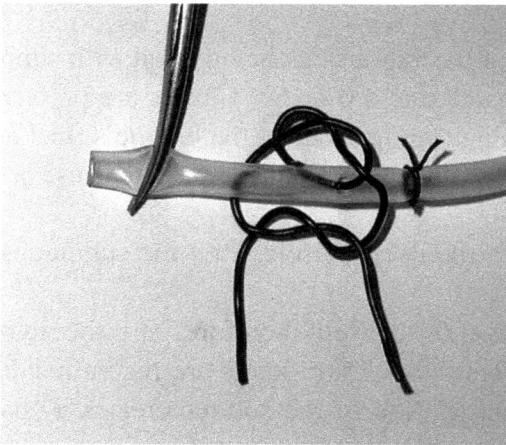

Figure 4.11 Stick suture applied to a large clipped vessel to arrest severe haemorrhage.

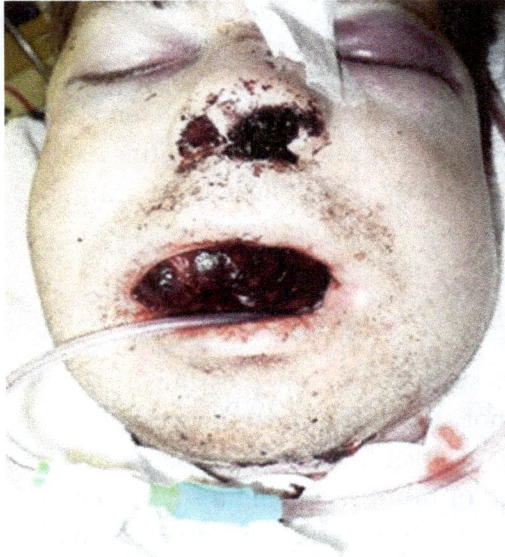

Figure 4.12   Persistent haemorrhage producing extensive oro-nasal swelling.

Tongue Wound Closure

- Small, linear lacerations can be repaired with simple interrupted sutures. Absorbable 4/0 or 5/0 sutures are preferred, with each suture passing through half of the tongue's thickness.
- For a tongue that is completely bisected, use a multi-layered closure.
- First, suture the deep muscle, then the submucosa, and finally the mucosa.
- The tongue tends to swell; therefore, care should be taken not to over-tighten sutures. Extra knots are recommended as frequent lingual manipulation of the sutures creates a chance of dehiscence.
- High-risk lacerations that require antibiotic prophylaxis include:
  o   heavily contaminated wounds and delayed presentation;
  o   immunocompromised individuals;

o   lacerations by animal or human bites;
o   ensuring both gram-positive and anaerobic antibiotic cover;
o   postoperative instructions emphasising a soft food diet.

Eyes and Eye Lids

- A laceration that involves the eyebrow should be re-approximated to recreate its natural curve. Leave the suture ends long to be easily distinguished from the eyebrow hairs. Do not shave the eyebrow as it may not grow back normally.
- For full-thickness eyelid injuries, the eyelid skin should be repaired loosely with 5/0 or 6/0 absorbable sutures. If the skin, muscle, tarsal plate, and underlying conjunctiva are severed, the conjunctiva does not need to be closed as a separate layer and will heal if the overlying tissues are well aligned.
- Start by placing a small suture (5/0 or 6/0) to approximate the grey line where the outer eyelid meets the inner conjunctiva i.e. the lash margin.
- Keep the knot away from the globe to avoid irritation of the conjunctiva or cornea.
- Use absorbable 5/0 sutures to approximate the tarsal plate and orbicularis muscle in one layer.
- Close the skin loosely with 5/0 or 6/0 simple absorbable sutures.
- Primary closure of the eyelid can be done with up to 25% full-thickness tissue loss. More than 25% full-thickness tissue loss requires complicated flaps.

Tear Duct Injuries

An injury to the tear duct (Figure 4.13) should be considered in any full-thickness eyelid laceration within 6 mm of the medial canthus which is where the upper and lower eyelids meet at the side of the nose. A tear duct injury can create a partial or complete obstruction to the drainage system. If tear duct probes and stents are available, the duct should be probed and possibly stented. As probing a tear duct is difficult, do not attempt without expert supervision.

Retrobulbar Haemorrhage and Orbital Compartment Syndrome

The orbit is a closed compartment, and infraorbital pressure can rise rapidly following a trauma-induced retrobulbar haemorrhage. The raised retrobulbar pressure needs to be released promptly to avoid irreversible optic nerve and retinal ischaemia which can occur within 60 min and cause permanent blindness within 1–2 h. The outcome is improved with immediate treatment by lateral canthotomy and inferior cantholysis (Figure 4.14) (see also Chapter 1, Skill station 3: Lateral canthotomy and cantholysis).

A blast war injury could cause globe rupture and loss of sight. This requires surgical enucleation of the globe and its replacement by an orbital prosthesis (Figure 4.15).

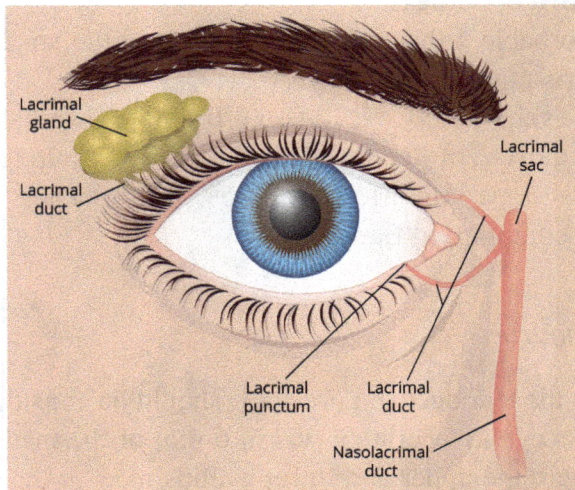

Figure 4.13   Lacrimal drainage system.

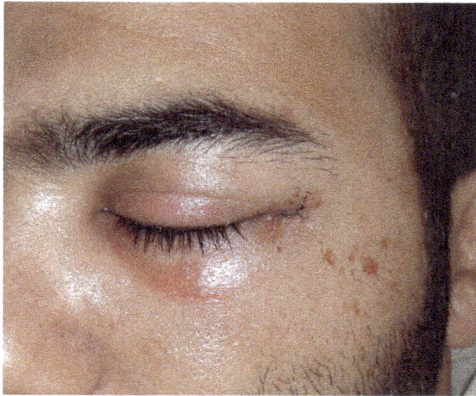

Figure 4.14 Retrobulbar pressure released by dividing the medial and lateral canthal tendon and its inferior branch — the crura (cantholysis), thus conserving sight.

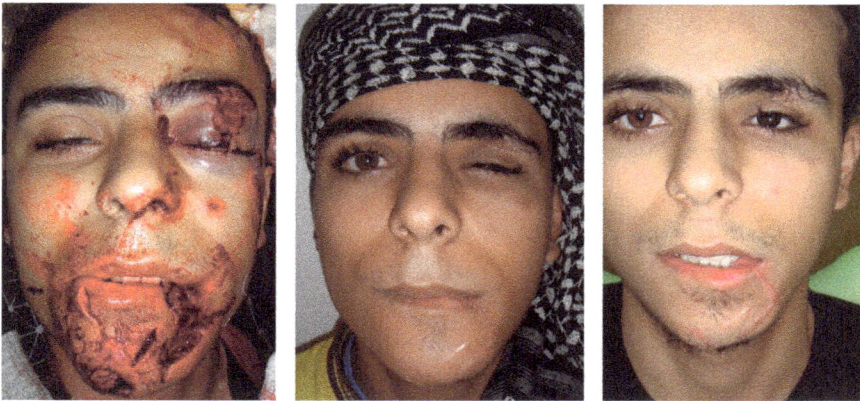

Figure 4.15 War injury, orbital perforation (left eye), replaced by orbital prosthesis.

Other Traumatic Causes of Orbital Proptosis

(1) Orbital emphysema is a self-limiting condition which results from forceful entry of air into the orbital soft tissue spaces due to facial trauma. As an example, orbital emphysema can be caused by forceful nose-blowing, although this is a rare occurrence.

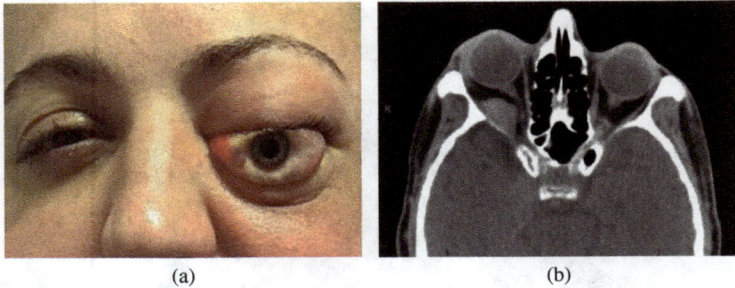

(a)   (b)

Figure 4.16   (a) Left orbital emphysema; (b) left orbital compartment syndrome, viewed from above.

Source: doi: 10.2147/OPTH.S180058. eCollection 2019. Dove Medical Press Ltd.

(2) An orbital blowout, unlike a *retrobulbar* haemorrhage (orbital compartment syndrome), may follow a fracture of the medial or inferior walls of the orbit due to the impact of a blunt object which causes emphysema (Figure 4.16).

(3) Proptosis can occur due to a skull base fracture with frontal lobe herniation into the orbit below. There is increased risk if the patient is taking anticoagulants.

Nasal Fractures

- A fractured nose often heals spontaneously within three weeks but if neglected, can leave a deformity.
- The correction may be carried out with bilateral infraorbital local anaesthetic infiltration with adrenaline or a general anaesthetic.
- Debride and clean the lesion, then manipulate any deformity. The nose has many blood vessels which results in epistaxis and requires packing.
- Nasal packing with petroleum jelly gauze should be performed carefully, especially if there is a possible anterior cranial fossa or orbital fracture with a cerebrospinal fluid (CSF) leak (Figure 4.17).
- Do not over pack to avoid fracture displacement. Stabilisation with a nasal splint has disadvantages, as superficial and full-thickness

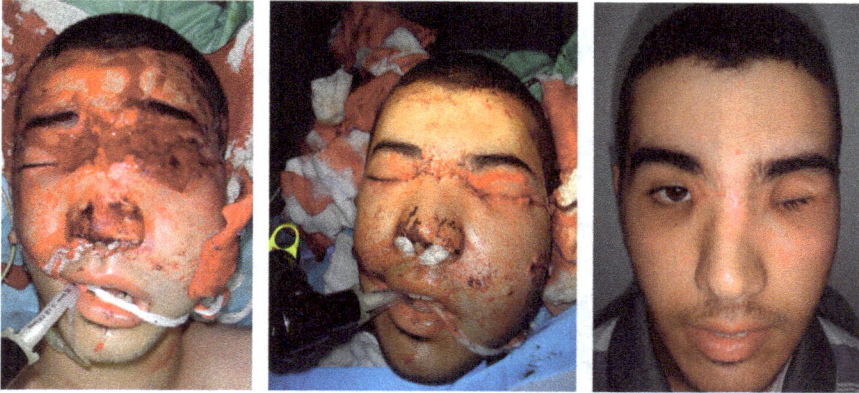

Figure 4.17   War injury with a comminuted nasal fracture and left global loss.

skin necrosis can occur if pressure is applied to the skin by a rigid splint. Distortion of the nose and instability can also occur.

- Use a 5/0 suture for the skin, but do not suture any cartilage.
- Carefully reduce any fracture and gently pack anteriorly with petroleum jelly gauze.
- Adhesive plaster (e.g. Micropore) provides adequate support (Figure 4.18).
- Provide analgesics, such as ibuprofen 400 mg six- to eight-hourly or diclofenac sodium 50 mg six-hourly.
- A rhinoplasty or septoplasty may be required after healing.

Beware of:
- a severe headache with blurred or double vision or difficulty in speaking which imply meningeal infection;
- a septal haematoma, which is a painful swelling obstructing breathing:
  - The septal haematoma needs to be drained and the nose packed with petroleum jelly gauze.
  - Two to three days later, remove the gauze.

If the septum's blood supply is cut off due to intranasal swelling, the cartilage within the nostrils can necrose giving a saddle nose. Also, beware of a clear nasal discharge suggesting a CSF leak.

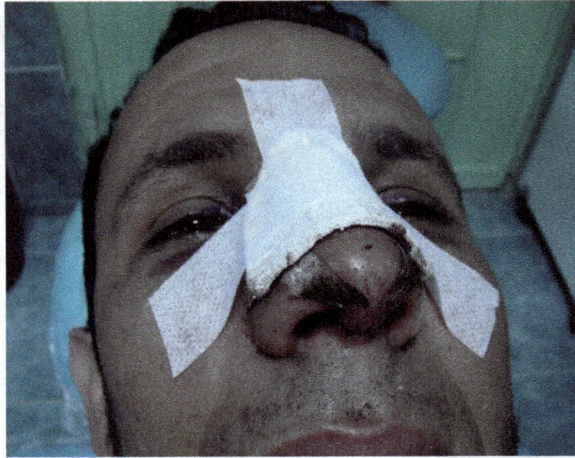

Figure 4.18   Simple splinting of a nasal fracture with adhesive paper tape rather than a rigid splint.

Nasal Bleeding (Epistaxis)

- To control bleeding from the nasal mucosa, apply 2% lignocaine with 1/200,000 adrenaline for local anaesthesia.
- Use absorbable 5/0 chromic sutures for the laceration.
- Once the repair is complete, loosely pack the affected nostril with povidone iodine gauze or petroleum jelly gauze. Leave the gauze in place for three days to encourage healing with less scar contracture.
- The patient will need analgesia, such as ibuprofen 400 mg six- to eight-hourly
- Primary repair of the internal nasal mucosa is challenging in a small, dark space. If the result is a tight intra-nasal scar, it may obstruct breathing (Figure 4.19).

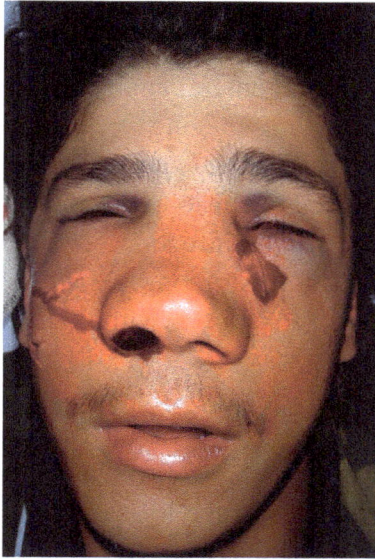

Figure 4.19   War injury with a comminuted nasal fracture, marked oedema and epistaxis.

Mandible, Maxilla, and Zygomatic Complex

Clinical Presentation

- Facial soft-tissue swelling and tenderness.
- Limited inter-incisor opening (trismus), malocclusion, and teeth tender or mobile on percussion.
- The temporomandibular joints are tender on palpation with trismus on attempted opening.
- Negative dental vitality test.
- Palpate the orbital margins and nose for tenderness and irregularities of underlying fractures.
- Facial sensory loss.
- Facial nerve paresis.

Treatment Goals

- Control of pain with parenteral analgesics.
- Obtain essential fracture imaging.
- Prepare and provide a general anaesthetic.
- Restore normal dental occlusion with intermaxillary fixation.
- Prevent or manage wound infection.
- Maintain nutrition and hydration.
- Control medication for patients with diabetes, hypertension, or other disorders.

Radiography

See Chapter 7 for examples of the following radiographic images:
- Appropriate periapical, occlusal, and bite-wing radiographs.
- Orthopantomographs (OPGs).
- Lateral skull and submental vertical radiographs.
- If available: computerised scans, magnetic resonance angiography (MRA), and magnetic resonance tomography (MRT).

Fracture Treatment

- Arrest haemorrhage, debride wounds, and apply temporary dressings.
- Remove mobile, non-vital, or decayed teeth especially at the fracture sites.
- Identify un-displaced fractures and mobile teeth that occlude.
- Carry out fracture reduction under a general or local anaesthetic and stabilise with intermaxillary fixation.
- Replace deficient blood, fluid, and intravenous electrolytes.
- Provide antibiotics and analgesics.
- Prescribe postoperative soft diet.
- Provide fluids at 1.5–2 litres a day.

Temporomandibular Joint (TMJ) Fracture Involving the Condylar Head and Neck

A TMJ fracture can be unilateral or bilateral. Unless displaced, treatment is unnecessary. In the case of extensive displacement, open reduction and fixation with a miniature plate is recommended.

Mandibular Fracture Stability

Intermaxillary fixation (IMF) is an important technique used to ensure the reduction and fixation of mandibular fractures. The type of IMF will be determined by the type of fracture. It is important to determine whether it is displaced or undisplaced (Figures 4.20 and 4.21).

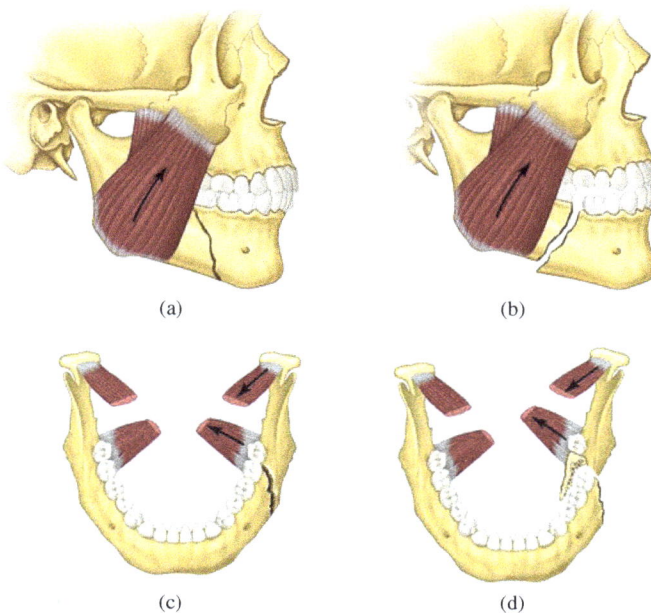

(a) (b)

(c) (d)

Figure 4.20 Mandibular angle fracture: (a) horizontally favourable; (b) horizontally unfavourable; (c) vertically favourable; (d) vertically unfavourable.

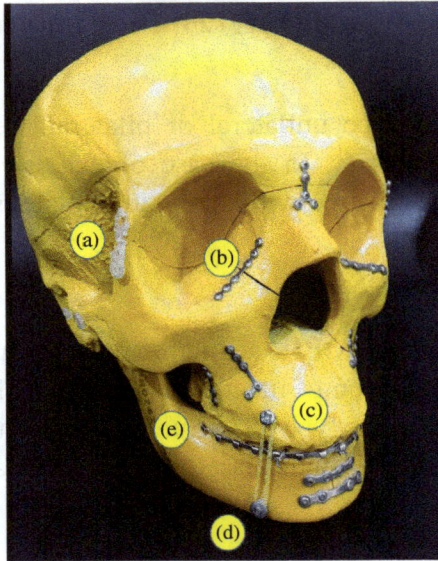

Figure 4.21   Model skull showing the reconstruction of a variety of maxillofacial fracture sites using osteosynthesis with miniaturised screwed plates: (a) absorbable plate; (b) malleable titanium plates; (c) and (d) IMF screws with a rubber band; (e) Erich arch bar, which requires a complimentary maxillary arch bar to achieve a stable dental occlusion.

There are many methods to achieve IMF, such as the Erich arch bar, dental eyelet wiring, IMF miniature plates and screws. Each technique has its own advantages. Chapter 1 focuses on two simple techniques — the Erich arch bar and dental eyelet wires — illustrating external pin fixation to achieve occlusal stability.[1,2]

Reduction and Intermaxillary Fixation Under General Anaesthetic Using Dental Eyelet Wiring

(Also see Chapter 1, Simulation Skill Stations 5 and 6 for detailed demonstrations).

The dental wiring technique has been implemented since World War I and is still reliable in austere environments with limited

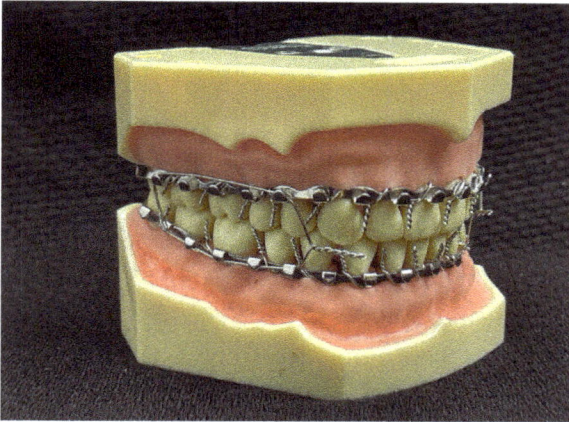

Figure 4.22 Intermaxillary fixation using Erich arch bars.[4,5] Stretched stainless-steel wire loops added to the cleats of the arch bars for intermaxillary fixation.

resources. If there is a simple fracture in either or both jaws, it is crucial that healthy teeth are available to articulate to each other and restore a normal dental occlusion. This technique is not useful if there are no teeth or if the present teeth cannot withstand the force required by fracture reduction because of severe periodontal disease. In such cases, dentures can be used to fix the alveolar fracture.

Eyelet wiring is a well-known technique implemented in austere environments for two reasons: high incidence of jaw fractures and its simplicity of use (Figure 4.22).

Favourable fractures may only need IMF for stabilisation, whereas unfavourable fractures (severe cases with loss of bony continuity) require reduction and interosseous wiring or screwed miniature plates for stabilisation. External pin fixation implemented for IMF is beyond the level of training presented in this chapter.

Classification of Maxillary Fractures

See Chapter 7 (Imaging) for explanation of Le Fort classification.

On Examination of Midface Fractures

Take note of:

- any malocclusion, consisting of an anterior open bite and mid-face mobility;
- the stability of the dentition and remove any dental fragments;
- facial asymmetry and palpate steps in the nasal dorsum and inferior orbital margins;
- the irregularity of the zygomatico-frontal suture area and zygomatic arch;
- impaired sensation of the maxillary nerves (VII and VIII);
- any intraoral ecchymosis.

Management

- Midface fractures are diagnosed by clinical examination revealing maxillary mobility and irregular intermaxillary articulation.
- OPG and 3-D computed tomography (CT) scans will complement periapical radiographs where possible.
- **With a general anaesthetic**, apply Rowe's disimpaction forceps to mobilise and restore the maxillary segment (Figure 4.23).
- The optimum means of internal fixation of midface fractures is with titanium or vitalium miniature plates and screws. The plates should be applied across the fracture lines.
- Initial airway patency must be confirmed by providing assisted ventilation with nasotracheal intubation or, in rare cases, with a tracheostomy.

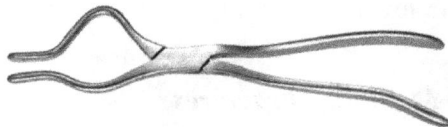

Figure 4.23   Rowe's disimpaction forceps.

- Leave the Erich arch bars on for one to two weeks in case training elastics are needed for any occlusal disharmony.
- The titanium and vitallium plates and screws are not removed.

Zygomatic Complex Fractures

The management of Zygomatic complex fractures (Figures 4.24 and 4.25) includes the following:

- Nondisplaced fractures do not require treatment.
- Depressed zygomatic complex fractures require elevation through a cutaneous/temporalis fascia incision above the hairline. If unstable, fix by exposure intraorally at the zygomaticofrontal junction with miniature plates and screws.[3]
- Depressed zygomatic arch can be simply elevated (Figure 4.24).

Facial Fractures in Children (Also See Chapter 5 Paediatric Surgery)

The healing process is quicker than in adults, but children have growth centres and active development needs to be ensured.

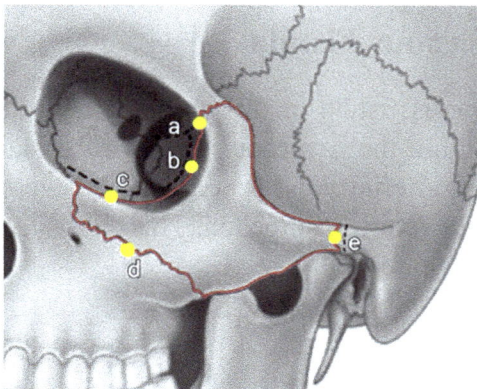

Figure 4.24   Zygomatic (malar) fractures. Potential zygomatic fracture sites are as follows: (a) fronto-zygomatic fracture; (b) and (c) orbital floor/zygomatic fractures; (d) zygomatic maxillary fracture; (e) zygomatic arch fracture.

Management of Non-Infected Dentoalveolar Fractures

Dentoalveolar fractures may be life threatening due to the inhalation of loose teeth. Therefore, it is important to examine the oral cavity for any dentoalveolar gaps so that avulsed teeth can be found, reinserted, and splinted (Figure 4.25).

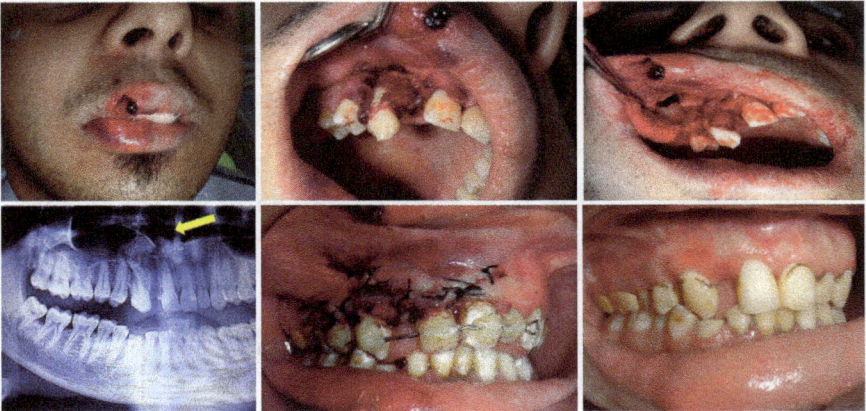

Figure 4.25   Use of composite cement with 0.5-mm wire to stabilise the avulsed upper-right first premolar, canine, and lost lateral incisor caused by a blast injury.

Carotid-Cavernous Fistula

A carotid-cavernous fistula results from an abnormal leak of the carotid artery within the cavernous sinus in the skull. The carotid blood under high arterial pressure enters the cavernous sinus, and the normal venous return is impeded. This causes a carotid-cavernous venous engorgement (Figure 4.26).

Clinical features: A bulging red pulsating eye, double vision or loss of vision, impaired eye movement, severe headaches, and nose bleeds.

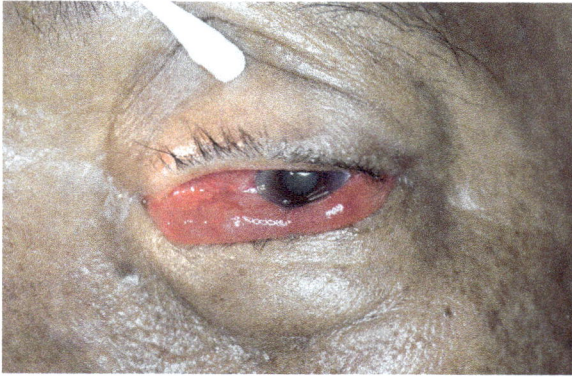

Figure 4.26 Internal carotid artery fistula bleeds into the cavernous sinus producing a bulging red eye. This is due to venous engorgement of the sinus.

Causes: Common causes of carotid-cavernous sinus fistula can be motor vehicle accidents, inter-personal violence, high blood pressure, and falls.

Investigations: CT, magnetic resonance imaging (MRI), ultrasound, and angiography.

Treatment: Placing platinum coils at the abnormal connection to separate artery blood flow from vein blood flow.

An Illustrative Case Study

A typical facial war trauma case, this patient was driving an open-topped car at night without lights. He collided with a broken-down tank, and the circle on his face shows the impact made by the end of the gun (Figure 4.27).

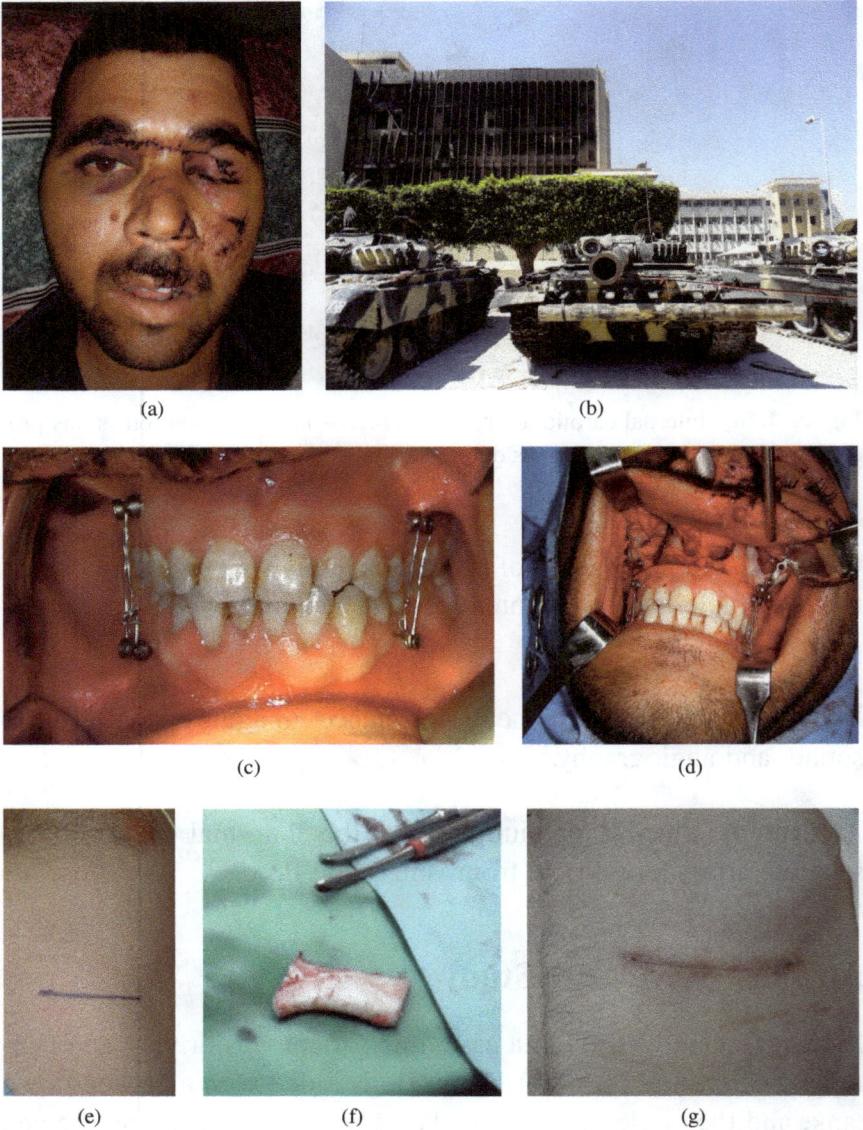

(a)   (b)

(c)   (d)

(e)   (f)   (g)

Figure 4.27   (a) Before treatment: Injuries sustained were Le Fort I fracture, orbital floor fracture of the left eye, fracture of the lateral wall of the orbital wall, left-upper eyelid soft tissue loss, and facial soft tissue injuries; (b) Broken-down tank; (c) Intermaxillary pin fixation; (d) Treatment of Le Fort I using plates, screws, and stainless-steel wire; (e–h) Enophthalmos correction: orbital

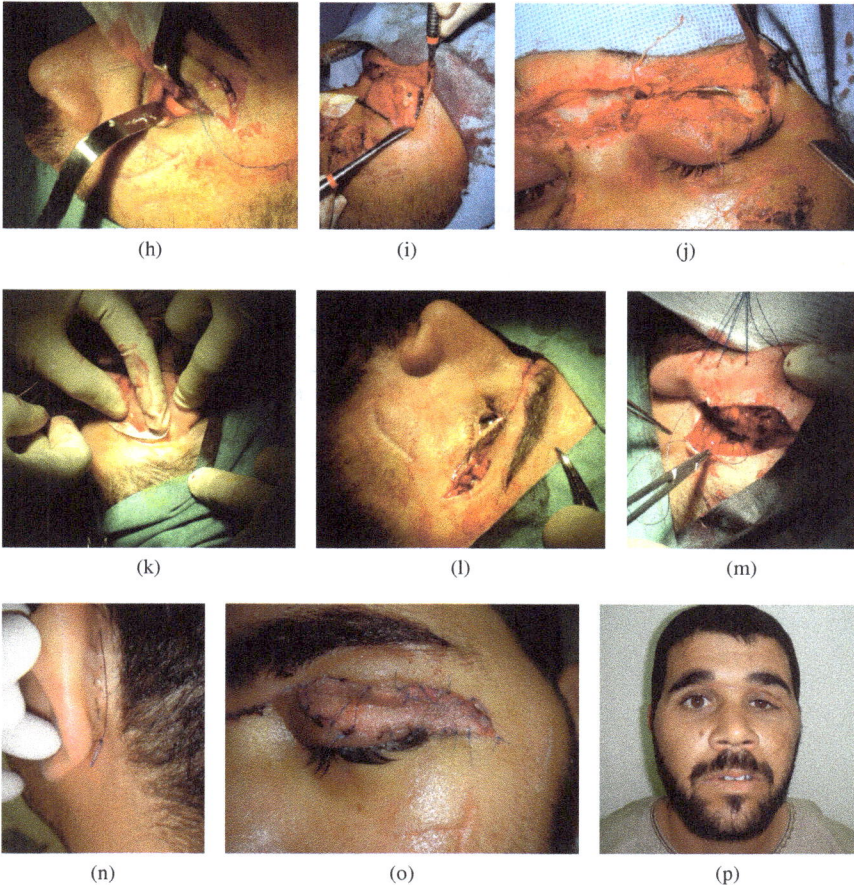

(h)   (i)   (j)

(k)   (l)   (m)

(n)   (o)   (p)

Figure 4.27 (*Continued*) floor treated using a costal cartilage graft harvested from the patient's eighth rib on the left side; (i) and (j) Shrapnel removed from upper eyelid, the wound cleaned, and the skin loss requires a graft; (k) Paper template is used to take the required skin for the graft from post auricular skin; (l) Suturing the skin graft in place; (m) Closing the ear donor site; (n) Healing ear, 10 days after the operation; (o) Healing upper eyelid graft, 10 days after the operation; (p) Follow up picture, after two months.

References

1. Falci SG, Douglas-de-Oliveira DW, Stella PE, Santos CR. Is the Erich arch bar the best intermaxillary fixation method in maxillofacial fractures? A systematic review. *Med Oral Patol Oral Cir Bucal.* 2015 Jul 1;20(4):e494–e499. doi: 10.4317/medoral.20448. PMID: 26034929; PMCID: PMC4523263.
2. Gibbons AJ, Mackenzie N, Breederveld RS. Use of a custom designed external fixator system to treat ballistic injuries to the mandible. *Int J Oral Maxillofac Surg.* 2011 Jan;40(1):103–105. doi: 10.1016/j.ijom.2010.08.001. Epub 2010 Sep 16. PMID: 20846823.
3. Zaggut A, Perry M. Do orbital floor plates adequately protect against serious secondary injury? *Br J Oral Maxillofac Surg.* 2019 Jul;57(6):539–542. doi: 10.1016/j.bjoms.2018.12.022. Epub 2019 May 16. PMID: 31104920.
4. Zaggut AW, Rahman MM, Youssef G, Holmes S, Ellamushi H, Shibu M, Ghanem A, Myers S, Harris M. Craniomaxillofacial war injuries in Misrata, Libya. *J Dent Open Access.* 2020 Aug. doi: 10.31487/j.JDOA.2020.02.05.
5. Zaggut AW, Rahman MM, Ghanem A, Myers S, Harris M. Training non-specialists for craniomaxillofacial trauma in a warzone setting. *J Dent Open Access.* 2020 Sep. doi: 10.31487/j.JDOA.2020.02.06.

Chapter 5

Paediatric Craniofacial Injuries

John H. Phillips, Ian Loh, and Sabah Kalamchi

Introduction

Craniofacial injuries in the paediatric population, between birth and 21 years of age, are complex surgical problems. The evolving variation in function, anatomy, and growth potential is compounded by the psychological effects of such injuries on a developing individual's personality, which makes treatment challenging.[1] The theatre of war further complicates matters as the same unfortunate individual is entangled in a different world. Children are vulnerable to more violent aetiologies, such as blast injuries, while caught in unstable regions with restricted logistics and austere resources. The approach to children who sustain these injuries must be augmented to take these factors into account.[2]

Although treatment aims are similar to those of treating adults, the approaches to the paediatric patient with facial trauma are different because of the changing anatomic variations in the craniofacial skeleton and the potential for long-term growth disturbance.

The objectives of this chapter are to describe how the variation in anatomy affects paediatric craniofacial fracture patterns and management, to highlight the effect war has on the approach to these injuries, and to provide guidelines for the reconstruction of these injuries in the setting of war.

Anatomical Differences

The growth and developmental differences of the paediatric craniofacial skeleton include the following:

(1) Growth ratio of the cranium to the face.
(2) Paranasal sinuses.
(3) Bone morphology and metabolism.
(4) Tooth buds.
(5) Fixation and growth.

Growth Ratio of the Cranium to the Face

At three months of age, the cranium-to-face ratio is 8:1, evolving to 4:1 by age two, and to 2.5:1 by age 5.5. At skeletal maturity, which is around age 16 for females and 21 for males, the ratio is 2:1 (Figure 5.1). This higher cranial-to-facial ratio translates to an increased likelihood of skull fractures and head injuries rather than facial fractures in the younger children. The proportional growth differences are due to the rapid growth of the neurocranium when compared to the facial

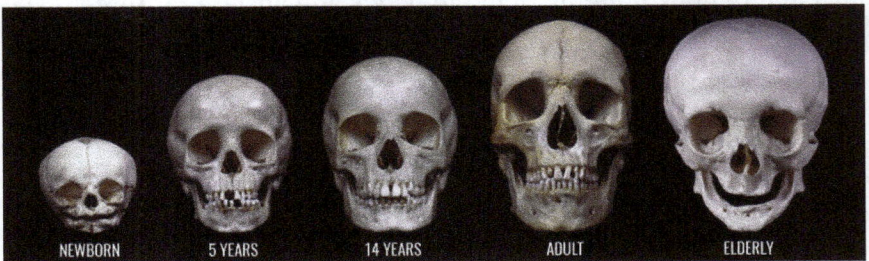

NEWBORN   5 YEARS   14 YEARS   ADULT   ELDERLY

Figure 5.1   Changing growth of the infantile oval-shaped cranium to the adolescent rectangular shape and finally the oval elderly cranium.

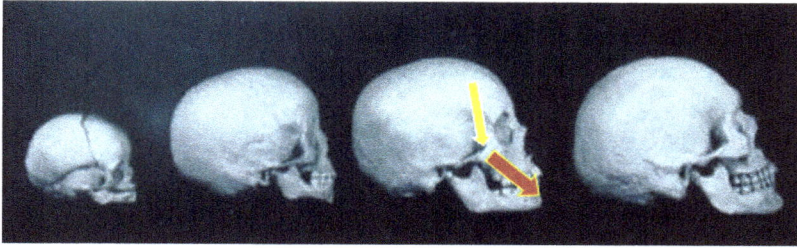

Figure 5.2 With age, the facial height (red arrow) grows downwards and forwards compared to the cranial height (yellow arrow).

skeleton.[3] The neurocranium is 75% complete at two years and 95% by the age of 10, whereas facial growth is only 65% complete at the age of 10. Cranial growth is dictated by the rapid underlying brain expansion (it triples in volume within the first 12 months) and driven from cranial sutures. Cranial growth slows after three years of age as the fontanelles close, sutures narrow over time, and fuse in adulthood.

Facial growth, on the other hand, follows a spasmodic trajectory until puberty due to multiple factors that include facial sutures, synchondrosis, and bone apposition and resorption. Facial dimensions steadily grow until roughly 80% complete at the age of five, then slow down until the onset of puberty, where hormonal influences mediate a second acceleration of growth to maturity. The disconnected maturation of facial growth is evident when comparing upper, middle, or lower facial development. The cranium and orbital growth are 95% completed growth by six to eight years of age and therefore the principles of adult facial trauma may be applied in these areas after this age. The maxilla and mandible however continue to grow until skeletal maturity (Figure 5.2).

Paranasal Sinuses

The maxillary sinuses are evident at four to five months, the ethmoids around 12 months, and frontal sinuses at six years of age (Figure 5.3).

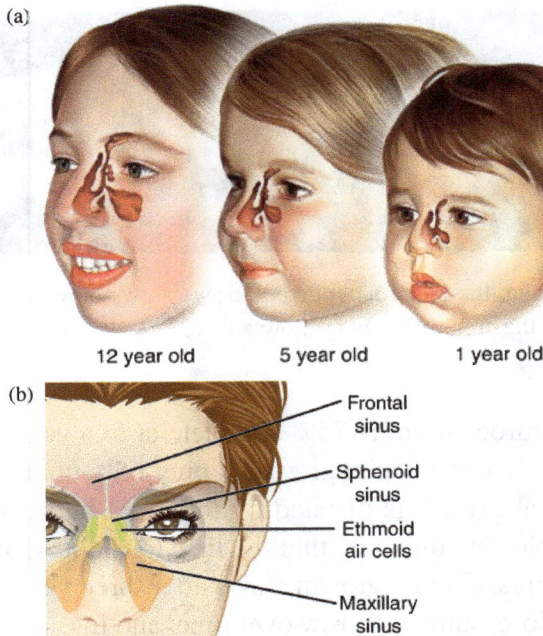

Figure 5.3   (a) Expansion of the growing facial air sinuses; (b) Four bilateral adult air sinuses.

Source: Image licensed under CC BY-SA 3.0. By OpenStax College, Anatomy & Physiology, Connexions Website. http://cnx.org/content/col11496/1.6/, Jun 19, 2013.

Bone Morphology and Metabolism

There is a significantly increased metabolism in children with faster fracture healing and therefore less time needed for immobilisation. In fractures of the mandible for instance, a child can be immobilised for two to three weeks with healing, whereas an adult usually requires six weeks of immobilisation (Figure 5.4). Children also have a greater cancellous-to-cortical ratio making them more elastic and resistant to deformation. There is a higher impact force per unit area needed for failure or displacement. Children however have a higher incidence of associated injuries when a fracture does occur.

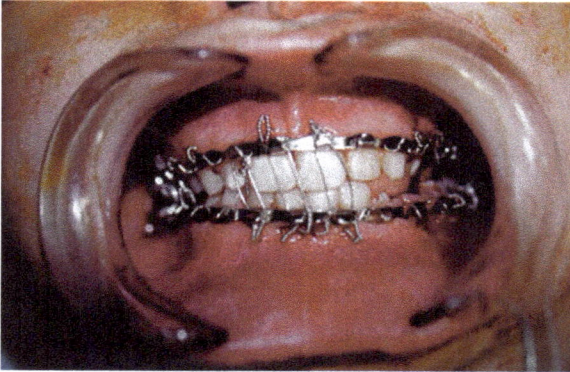

Figure 5.4   Intermaxillary fixation in a child requires a shorter period of immobilisation than in adults.

As the facial skeleton matures, increasingly mineralised and pneumatised, the incidence of facial fractures rises. Paediatric patients are more likely to develop greenstick fractures and present with oblique craniofacial fracture patterns due to the elasticity of their bone. The typical Le Fort fracture patterns are not commonly seen in the younger patients.

Tooth Buds

Evolving dentition with the presence of uninterrupted tooth buds increases bone strength. Tooth growth can be divided into three separate groups:

- Primary dentition (0–5 years)
- Mixed dentition (6–11 years)
- Permanent dentition (12–16 years)

Mixed dentition can also make the process of applying arch bars more difficult because of loose teeth in this age group. A higher tooth-to-bone ratio equates to weaker bone and therefore in the mixed dentition group, there is increased incidence of maxillary and mandibular fractures.

Fixation and Growth

The presence of a smaller body mass and thicker, soft tissues is protective in the paediatric patient.

Care must be taken in internal fixation approaches in children to monitor the need for removal as soon as healing occurs and the potential for growth restriction with time. Therefore, simple techniques for reduction and fixation with minimal periosteal stripping, such as the use of K-wire fixation and arch bars and intermaxillary fixation (IMF) may be an advantage in the paediatric population.

Epidemiology/Aetiology

Paediatric facial fractures are uncommon, accounting for only 4–9.2% of all fractures below the age of 16 in the Western world.[4] The distribution of facial fractures in the paediatric population is varied and age and gender dependent. Young males are twice to three times more likely to sustain a facial fracture when compared to young females.

Only 1% of all facial fractures occurred in children under the age of six years. This low incidence in children under the age of six years can be attributed to the high supervision and protected environments that toddlers and infants are afforded. This is not the case for children in a war environment. From the age of five or six years, rapid neuromotor development occurs and children begin to partake in riskier activities (Figure 5.5).

As the paediatric patient ages, there is a superior to inferior shift in the pattern fracture due to the decreasing cranial-to-facial ratio. The infant or younger child is more likely to sustain a frontal skull or orbital fracture, whereas children older than seven years of age are prone to maxillary, nasal, or mandibular fractures due to the increased prominence of these regions.

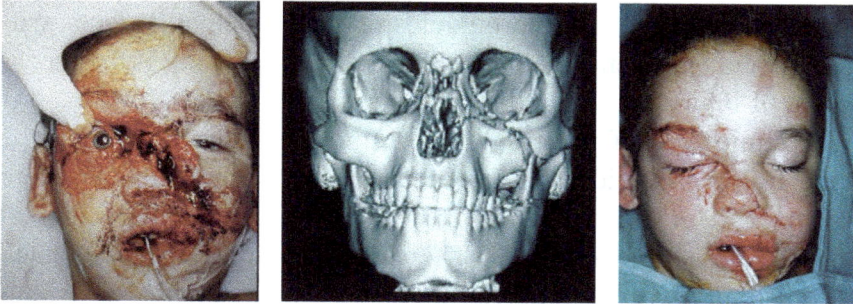

Figure 5.5   Five-year-old frontal bone fracture and midface laceration.

Fractures in younger patients were caused by falls or motor vehicle accidents, whereas older patients sustained fractures as a result of violence, assault, sports, or motor vehicle accidents. In the paediatric population, 73–88% of presentations had associated injuries, such as complex head injuries, skull fractures, ocular and soft-tissue involvement. Cervical spine, thoracic, and abdominal injuries are less common in this age group.[4]

The 3-D computed tomography (CT) scan shows fractures of the right orbit, nasal bones, and left zygomatico-maxillary suture.

A review of war injuries revealed that over two million children have died as a result of conflict and more than six million paediatric injuries have been documented.[5] Half of these injuries were either ocular, orbital, or craniofacial trauma. In Iran and Iraq, paediatric war victims accounted for 4–7% of admissions to US military hospitals, reflecting major resource costs. This patient population was also admitted for longer periods of time and had more complex recovery versus adults. Paediatric injuries from war made up 25% of inpatient hospital stay during the war in Afghanistan and 10% in Iraq.

Diagnosis

Diagnosis of facial fractures in the paediatric population is challenging as it is common to have an uncooperative child coupled with anxious parents. A thorough history from patient, parents, witnesses, and emergency personnel can help in deducing if the mechanism of injury may have caused a facial fracture.

Examination of the child may require sedation but should be done following guidelines for emergency management of severe trauma and in tandem with emergency physicians. The cervical spine examination is crucial. There is a reported 10% associated risk of injury with craniofacial trauma.[6] A neurosurgical consultation should be considered as almost half of patients with facial fractures have concomitant neurological injuries. The patient's airway should be assessed urgently as midface or mandibular fractures as well as cervical spine injuries can complicate endotracheal intubation. Anaesthetic support may be required to establish a non-surgical airway as the tongue is proportionally larger in the paediatric population than in adults and predisposes to airway obstruction.

Examination should start by observation of the patient's overall condition followed by a top-down ordered assessment. Palpation of the skull for wounds, haematoma, or deformity signifying an underlying skull fracture. Examine the supraorbital ridge and frontal bone, assess for paraesthesia of the supra-orbital nerve. In patients without frontal sinuses, these fractures are basically anterior base of skull fractures.

Orbital examination follows and is extremely important due to the high risk of ocular and periorbital injury (globe rupture, orbital apex syndrome, superior orbital fissure syndrome, corneal abrasions, entrapped extra-ocular muscles, lacrimal drainage system laceration, and medial canthal avulsions). Subconjunctival haemorrhage is characteristic of an orbital fracture as the conjunctiva is related to the orbital periosteum. Nasal examination begins with palpation of the nasal root caudally, examining for nasal deviation, nasal dorsal compressibility, signs of cerebrospinal fluid (CSF) rhinorrhoea, and intra-nasal examination for septal haematoma with a speculum.

Midface examination begins with palpation of the orbital rims, checking for a step deformity, cheek paraesthesia (infra-orbital nerve) and palpation of the zygoma (look for loss of malar prominence and lateral canthal dystopia). Midface stability can be tested by manual distraction of the maxilla whilst anchoring the head. This is best done under sedation. Check for hemotympanum or base of skull fracture (mastoid haematoma — Battle's sign).

Occlusion should be assessed as the examination transitions to the mandible; a subjective malocclusion is a sensitive sign that there is a mid to lower facial fracture. Although patients with mixed dentition may have pre-existing malocclusion, open bites or maligned dental arches are indicative of a mandibular fracture. Examine for missing or loose teeth, palpate the mandible from the Temporomandibular joint (TMJ) to symphysis for any signs of pain.

Diagnostic imaging is essential in the evaluation of facial fractures. Computed tomography (CT) scan of the skull to mandible with coronal, axial, and 3-D reconstructions are the gold standard. A panoramic radiograph may also be useful to visualise mandible fractures.

Paediatric Craniofacial War Injuries

Craniofacial war injuries are seen in 25–40% of battlefield casualties even though the head and neck region account for only 12% of body surface area. Advances in medical resuscitation in the setting of war and changes in the type of warfare have seen an increase in treatable craniofacial trauma.

Data from the wars in Iraq and Afghanistan paint a picture of the type of head and neck injuries sustained by children during the conflict:

Face and cheek 48%, neck larynx and trachea 18%, mouth and lip 12%, eyelid 4%, nose 3%, and ear 2%. The majority of craniofacial fractures during the two conflicts were maxillary-mandibular fractures (25–72%) and frontal bone fractures (33%). The incidence of other facial bone fractures in the paediatric population were max-illa 25%, mandible 21–72%, zygomatic-orbit 19%, teeth 13%, and nose 12%.

Children, who are often caught in the middle of a conflict, lack protective clothing such as helmets, armoured vests, or protective eyewear. The aetiologies of their injuries are mainly blast injuries from improvised explosive devices (IEDs), gunshots, burns, or motor vehicle accidents. The majority of trauma seen by surgeons in the Western world is caused by low-velocity energy incidents, but the injuries sustained in war, as seen in Afghanistan, are due to high-energy exchange trauma causing extensively contaminated and com-minuted displaced fractures with associated soft-tissue avulsion.

The blast effect on children is different when compared to an adult due to their greater skeletal elasticity but decrease in tensile and compressive strengths. The increased skeletal elasticity trans-lates to an increase in shear injuries due to the critical shear stresses behind the front of a compressive shock wave (Friedlander wave). Concomitant complex head injuries are seen more regularly in the paediatric cohort because the thinner calvarium makes the brain more vulnerable to blast wave effects and penetrating injuries. Paediatric patients are also predisposed to rapid upper airway obstruction due to the anatomical difference in the location of the glottis (more superior and anterior in relation to the pharynx) and greater tongue proportion.

Increased risk of infection from contaminated IEDs, secondary low-pressure wave of the blast effect sucking dirt into the wound, and delays in treatment add further complexity to an already diffi-cult situation.

Treatment of Paediatric Craniofacial War Injuries

The modern initial management of these injuries depends on the mechanism of injury and the overall severity of the injuries sus-tained by the patient. The priorities are to save life, secure airway, save vision, salvage limbs, and then to give the best functional and aesthetic outcome for other wounds.

Emergency procedures such as intubation, cricothyroidotomy, or lateral canthotomy should be performed to secure the airway, especially in children under the age of 12, or to decompress an impending orbital apex or superior orbital fissure syndrome. Children have a superior functional reserve and can maintain a stable heart rate and blood pressure for a longer period of time before suddenly deteriorating. To avoid this, bleeding points should be compressed, large bore intravenous access acquired, and resuscitation commenced prior to evacuation.

All wounds should be irrigated and surgically debrided judiciously once the patient is stabilised and safely evacuated from the site of trauma/battlefield. Surgical debridement should aim to clean and stabilise the wound to prevent infection; this should be done in serial procedures until the wound is clean. The most common procedures performed in the paediatric population are[6]:

- complex facial lacerations with multiple-layer repair to decrease dead space (up to one-third of all procedures);
- airway procedures, including tracheostomy or cricothyroidotomy (up to 25%);
- neck exploration for penetrating neck trauma (up to 13%);
- arch bars or K-wire fixation mandible;
- open reduction internal fixation (ORIF) other facial fractures;
- burns management;
- craniotomy.

Procedures to Teach

Concept of Irrigation and Debridement of Facial Lacerations

Facial lacerations vary depending on the mechanism of injury, location, size, composite depth, and associated structures involved.

Regardless of the complexity, all wounds must be thoroughly irrigated with normal saline or water, assessed, and appropriately debrided. This helps to prevent infection and haematoma formation and remove debris or non-viable tissue from the wound.

To maintain the aesthetic of the face, debridement should be minimised to maximise tissue preservation and achieve primary closure where possible. Granick et al. describe a useful classification for debridement based on the Jackson burn wound model, where the necrotic centre is bordered by a marginal area of potentially viable tissue which in turn is surrounded by healthy tissue.[7] The classification is described according to the level of debridement.

Classification of Debridement

Debridement	Nondebrided	Incomplete	Marginal	Complete	Radical
Code	0	1	2	3	4

Incomplete debridement leaves residual necrotic tissue, and this is to be avoided if possible as there is an increased risk of infection and inflammation. Marginal debridement is desired, where all necrotic tissue is removed but potentially viable tissue remains after the initial surgery. Removing more tissue at the initial debridement than is necessary will equate to an unnecessary larger wound requiring more complicated reconstruction in an already complex patient.

Layered Wound Closure

Wherever possible, facial lacerations should primarily be sutured in well-approximated layers. Deep lacerations with fascial and muscle involvement require exploration and repair of special structures, such as sensory and motor nerves, the parotid duct, and lacrimal drainage system. Muscle and fascia should be approximated with fine absorbable suture, such as Vicryl or Monocryl. Special structures may require repair under loupe or microscopic magnification. Repairing the muscular and subcutaneous layers ablates dead space that could lead to haematoma or infection. The dermis should also be repaired in layers using buried interrupted deep dermal sutures to decrease skin tension and prevent scar widening.

Approach to the Emergency Paediatric Surgical Airway

Severe facial trauma may present with the life-threatening situation of 'can't intubate, can't oxygenate (CICO)', especially in the chaos of a war zone. The ability to secure an emergent surgical airway in the CICO situation is vital in the resuscitation and stabilisation of the child. The available surgical airway techniques can be divided into needle based: percutaneous cannula cricothyroidotomy (PCC) or trans-tracheal jet ventilation and scalpel based: surgical cricothyroidotomy or tracheostomy.

The age of the patient is an important factor in choosing which technique to perform due to anatomical differences in the paediatric airway. The Difficult Airway Society (www.das.uk.com) recommends PCC if there is no ear, nose, or throat surgeon available to perform a surgical tracheostomy; however, the literature suggests that in children under the age of eight, surgical cricothyroidotomy or tracheostomy should be considered. This is because, apart from the known complications of PCC (surgical emphysema, pneumothorax, and interstitial lung injury), children have a smaller trachea and short, wide necks that prevent the operator from achieving the correct angle of approach to cannulate the trachea — the steeper the angle, the higher the risk of posterior tracheal wall injury.

Furthermore, surgical cricothyroidotomy should be performed with extreme care as the size of the cricothyroid membrane in younger children is much narrower; also, the thyroid cartilage can be hidden by the more prominent hyoid and cricoid cartilages.

Burn Injury and Wound Care

Burn injury is inevitable in the setting of war due to the blast- and thermal-type injuries. Basic first-aid treatment provided immediately can dramatically improve the degree of injury. This includes immediate removal from the burn stimulus, removing clothing, and cooling of the affected areas with cool, running water (12–18°C).

Following adequate first aid, the initial assessment to direct management of the paediatric facial burn should include:

(1) confirmation of the burn injury mechanism;
(2) assessment of the extent of the burn — total body surface area (TBSA) %;
(3) determination of the depth of the burn injury.

Crystalloid intravenous resuscitation should be administered if the TBSA is >10% full-thickness burn, >20% TBSA mixed depth of burn or if the patient is one year old or younger as the smaller child is more susceptible to the systemic inflammatory response to burn injury. The modified Parkland formula (4 ml × kg × TBSA%) is used to calculate the required resuscitation volume, with half of the volume given in the first eight hours and the subsequent volume over the following 16 hours. In addition to this calculated volume, maintenance IV fluid containing sodium should be administered to prevent a hyponatraemic state from over-secretion of antidiuretic hormone. In children younger than one year of age, maintenance fluid should include dextrose (D5 + 1/2 NS) to prevent hypoglycaemia as their glycogen stores are easily depleted. Ongoing fluid requirements can be calculated based on urine output, aiming for a rate of 0.5–1.0 ml/kg/h.

Once the patient is stabilised and adequate analgesia has been provided, the burn injury itself can be cleaned, loose skin or blisters can be debrided, and the appropriate dressing applied. In the case of facial burns, dressings can be difficult to apply even without the interferences of concurrent wounds and airway support. Therefore, topical ointments, such as Flamazine or Polysporin, that minimise bacterial contamination, provide an optimal wound environment (moist) and promote re-epithelialisation, can be applied and if needed, reinforced with light gauze and net dressings. Depending on the choice of ointment, the burn injury can be cleaned and ointment reapplied daily or multiple times a day until the burn injury demarcates, and a decision can be made if burn debridement is necessary.

Treatment of Facial Fractures

Zygomatic Fractures

The incidence of isolated zygomatic fractures in children is low but increases when associated with orbital fractures and increasing age.[8] The zygoma is relatively resilient to fracturing in younger patients, where the immature maxillary sinus allows the zygomaticomaxillary buttress to dissipate force energy. If enough force is transmitted, the fracture dislocation pattern is oblique and occurs through the zygomaticofrontal suture, displacing the zygoma and orbital floor inferiorly.

Goals of treatment for paediatric zygomaticomaxillary fractures are to restore pre-injury facial appearance, preventing orbital dysmorphology (enophthalmos or vertical dystopia), and malocclusion. Non or minimally displaced fractures can be treated conservatively and closely followed up, but displaced fractures should undergo open reduction and internal fixation.

Fracture reduction is aimed at alignment of the lateral orbital wall, zygomaticofrontal suture, orbital rim, and zygomaticomaxillary buttress. The lateral orbital wall is the most accurate gauge of adequate reduction. Fixation can be achieved with titanium plating systems or in the absence of these sets, Kirschner wire (K-wire) fixation can be used.

K-wire fixation utilises a 2-mm stab incision over the affected malar eminence after reduction and fixation (intra-osseous wire or plate fixation) of the zygomaticofacial suture or lateral orbital wall. A 1.5-mm K-wire is passed medially through the deep portion of the main fractured zygomatic fragment horizontally. The K-wire is sent through the maxillary bone and nasal septum, and the tip is left in the contralateral maxillary sinus. An external K-wire of equal length can be placed over the patients face to gauge the final placement of the wire. The wire is then buried under the skin and removed after four weeks (Figure 5.6).

Mandibular Fractures: Establishing Occlusion and Arch Bars

The anatomical prominence of the mandible predisposes this bone to fracture from blunt force trauma. Mandibular fractures are the most common facial fractures reported in children over the age of

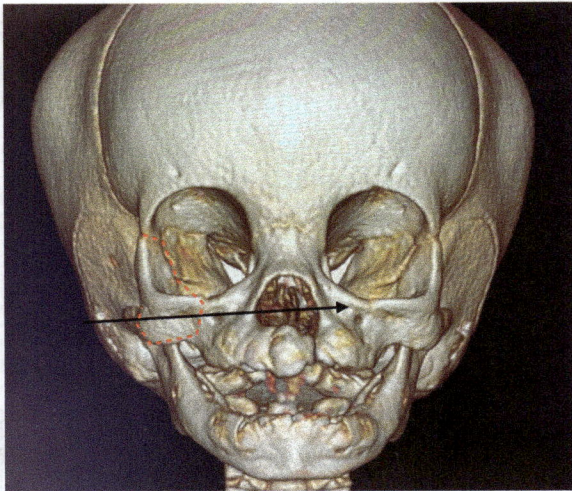

Figure 5.6   Direction of K-wire placement: frontal zygomatic maxillary fracture shown as the fine dotted red line through the lateral aspect of the orbit and inferiorly through the anterior maxilla.

six years. Paediatric mandibular fractures are more likely to be greenstick fractures or have long irregular sagittal patterns.

The goals for treatment include restoration of normal occlusion, to ensure bony union, and to avoid infection. Fixation of mandibular and even maxillary fractures can be difficult due to developing dental follicles and often a conservative approach is adopted i.e. soft diet, dental hygiene, and mandibular rest. Minor malocclusions are well tolerated in infants and younger children because of their enhanced ability to remodel fractures and have secondary orthodontic corrections to achieve a normal bite. Displaced fractures with significant malocclusion however require either open or closed reduction and a form of fixation.

In the absence of plating systems, arch bars or IMF screws can be utilised to achieve maxillary mandibular fixation (MMF) and immobilisation of the jaw to allow fracture healing. Once reduced and occlusion restored by checking occlusal contact points along the maxillary and mandibular dental arches, an upper and lower arch bar can be secured using 26-gauge stainless-steel wire loops to each tooth. The course of MMF usually lasts for two to three weeks, and the arch bars are removed once bony union is achieved.

Awareness of Ocular Injuries Including Debridement and Possible Globe Rupture and Need for Enucleation to Prevent Sympathetic Ophthalmoplegia

Penetrating Head Injuries

Ten percent of all trauma cases in children included the head. Of the head injuries, up to 70% involved penetrating head trauma of which one-third were children under the age of 15. The aim is to prevent wound infection and the treatment or prevention of a critical rise in intracranial pressure. The treatment in these cases involves the excision and debridement of clot, necrotic brain, and any left-behind fragments of missile or bone fragments. Other decisions include

whether to close the dura or not, to replace bone fragments or craniotomy bone depending on brain swelling and high intracranial
pressure, and the debridement and closure of the scalp to decrease
the risk of infection.

Conclusion

The matter of paediatric injuries in war should be unfathomable to
all of us; however, to quote the anti-war activist Widad Akreyi, *'Our
lives and the lives of future generations do not only depend on the
conflicts that take place but also on the solutions we offer in
response to them'.*

*'We need to decide that we will not go to war, whatever reason
is conjured up by the politicians or the media, because war in our
time is always indiscriminate, a war against innocents, a war
against children'* Howard Zinn.

Examples of Clinical Cases

Case 1

A six-month-old baby sustained a blast injury in the face in March
2011. The whole family was seriously injured or killed. There was
soft-tissue injury and bilingual bony fracture. The child arrived at
the field hospital at midnight, with no family support and no nursing
staff available.

Loss of tissue at the right commission later required revision
surgery to improve mouth opening and speech. Again, loss of soft
tissue of the upper-right eyelid later required revision surgery to
improve closure and prevent eye dryness and avoid infection.

The screws were positioned with care to avoid damaging the
follicles of the deciduous and permanent teeth. Although not an
issue in this particular case, it is important to protect the growth

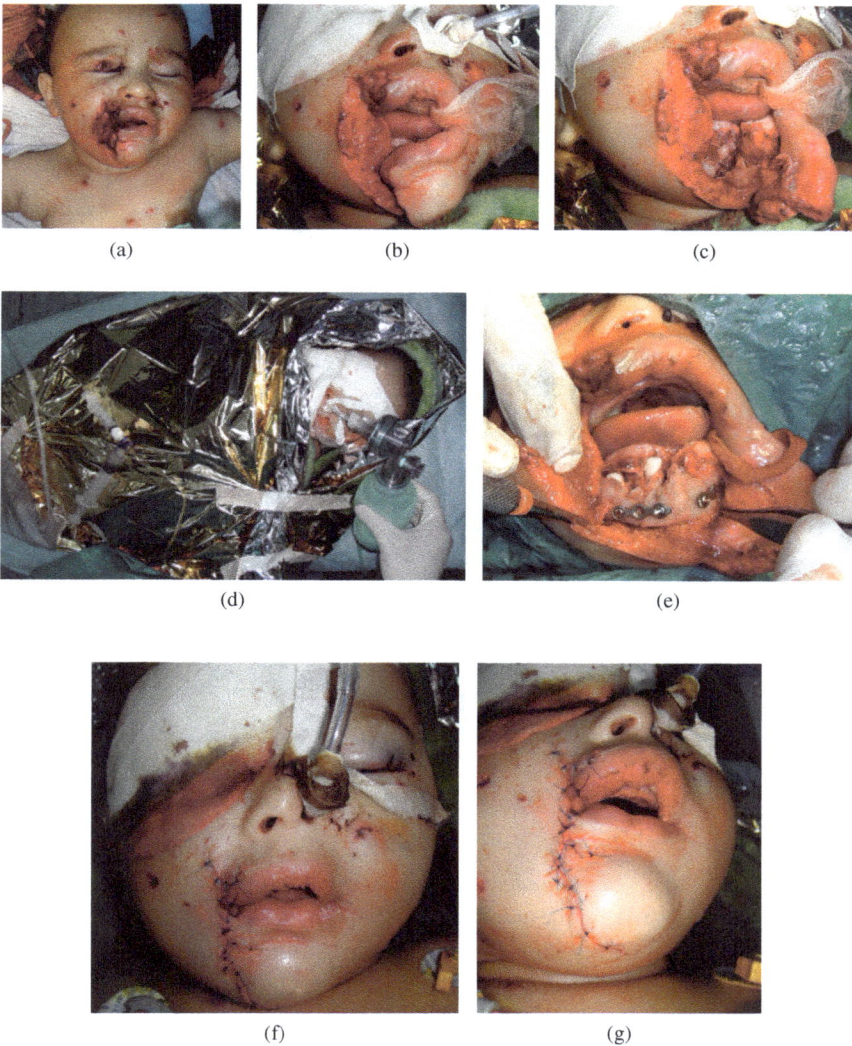

Figure 5.7 Case 1: (a–c) Injured baby on arrival at a field hospital in 2011; (d) Baby wrapped in a reflective blanket to protect him from the cold; (e) Mandibular fracture was fixed with adult screws and plates (which were the only ones available); (f) and (g) Immediate post-operative pictures.

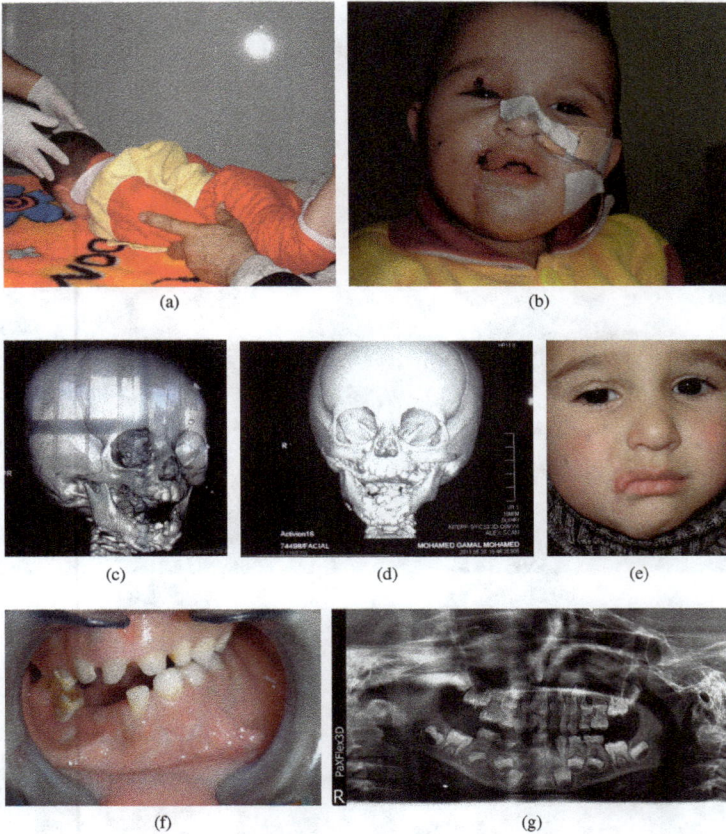

Figure 5.8   Case 1 (*Continued*): (a) Plain X-ray was taken next (the only type of scan available); (b) At the two-week follow up, with a nasogastric tube for feeding; (c–e) Eight weeks after initial treatment; Follow up in 2016. (f) Intraoral examination shows the fracture has fully healed; (g) OPG follow up confirms the bony healing and shows that the mixed dentition is healthy;

centres in the TMJ area because damage to them may distort the future development of the face (see Figure 5.7).

The baby was evacuated to Egypt, and the scans and the photo in Figure 5.8(c–e) were taken eight weeks after the initial treatment, when the screws and plates were removed.

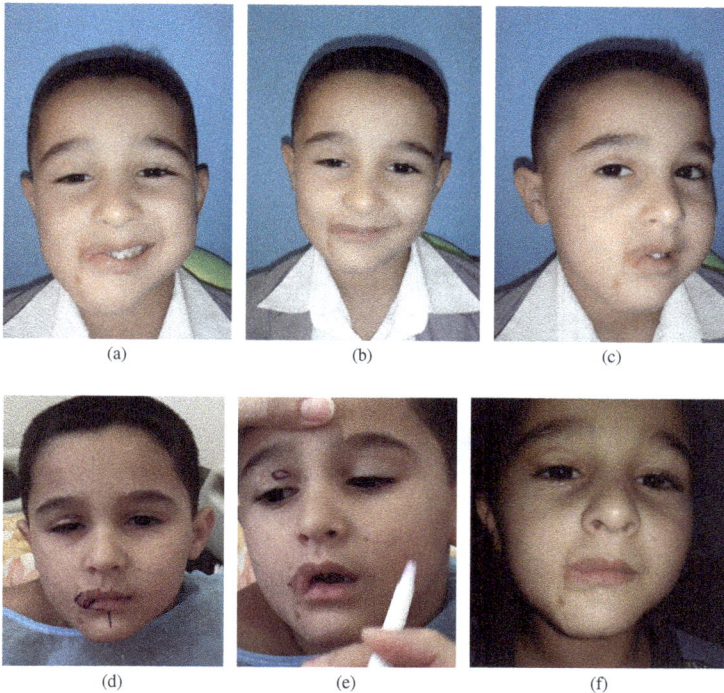

Figure 5.9 Case 1 Follow up in 2016, continued: (a–c) The child complained of limited mouth opening which affected his speech. Also, his eyelid didn't close properly; (d) and (e) Pre-operative site marking in preparation for the revision surgery on the lips and upper-right eyelid; (f) Post-operative frontal photograph showing follow up with maintenance of natural commissure appearance and function.

Case 2

A five-year-old suffered a left condylar fracture after a fall, but the diagnosis was missed probably because the dentist did not take an X-ray of the TMJ area (Figure 5.9). Later, her mother noticed that she developed mouth opening limitation, pain, and mouth opening deviation. Her case will be followed up as she grows to monitor the TMJ recovery.

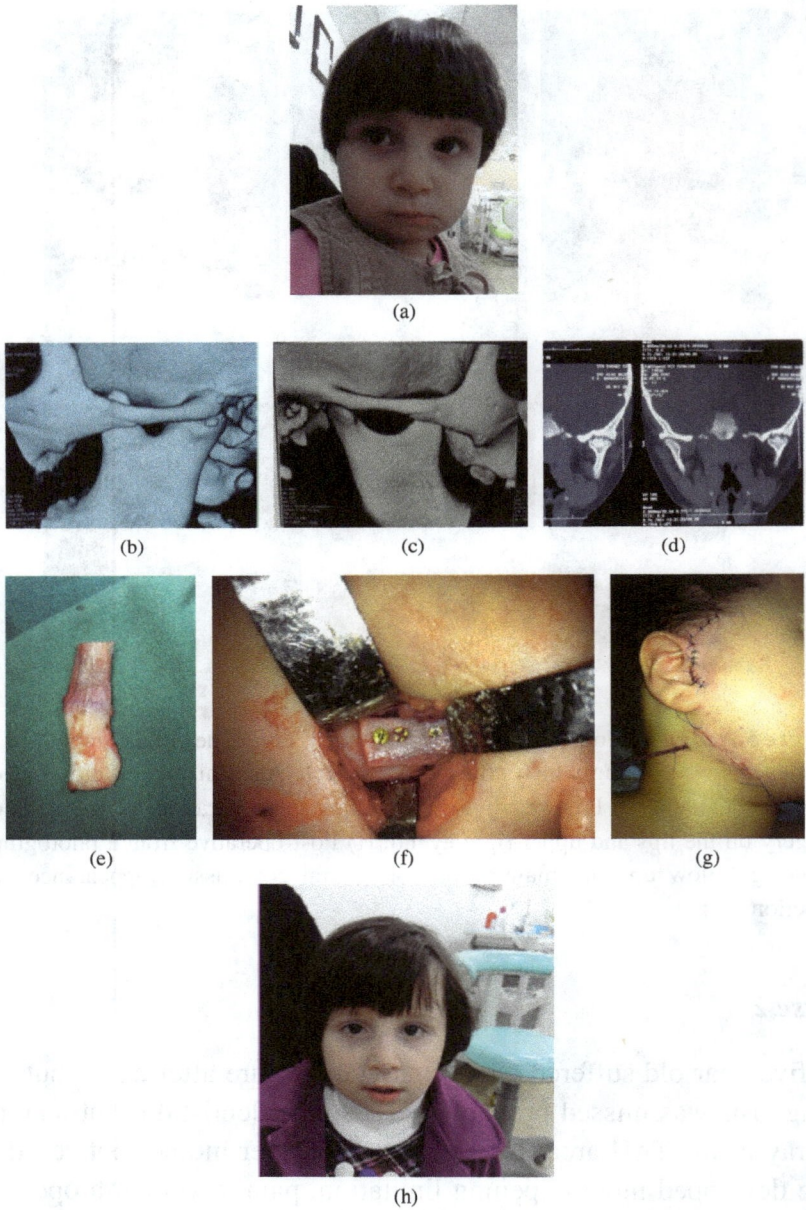

Figure 5.10   Case 2: (a–d) About two months after the original injury, the child was seen by an oral maxillofacial surgeon and an axial CT scan confirmed that the left condyle was ankylosed; (e–g) Child was treated with a costochondral graft; (h) Post surgery, the symptoms improved.

Case 3

This asymmetrical facial deviation to the left is the consequence of an inadequately treated fractured left mandible. It could be corrected at this stage with an osteotomy (Figure 5.11).

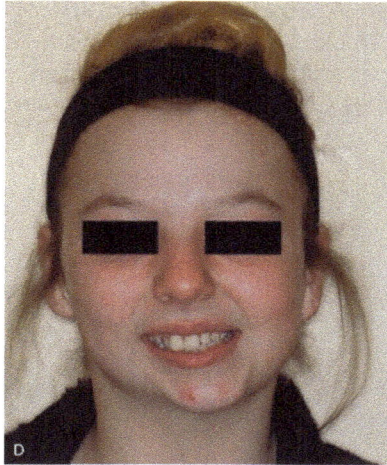

Figure 5.11　Case 3: Asymmetrical facial deviation.

References

1.　Morrow BT, Samson TD, Schubert W, Mackay DR. Evidence-based medicine: Mandible fractures. *Plast Reconstr Surg.* 2014 Dec;134(6):1381–1390. doi: 10.1097/PRS.0000000000000717. PMID: 25415101.
2.　Steed MB, Schadel CM. Management of pediatric and adolescent condylar fractures. *Atlas Oral Maxillofac Surg Clin North Am.* 2017 Mar;25(1):75–83. doi: 10.1016/j.cxom.2016.10.005. PMID: 28153186.
3.　Smartt JM Jr, Low DW, Bartlett SP. The pediatric mandible: I. A primer on growth and development. *Plast Reconstr Surg.* 2005 Jul;116(1):14e–23e. doi: 10.1097/01.prs.0000169940.69315.9c. PMID: 15988242.
4.　Imahara SD, Hopper RA, Wang J, Rivara FP, Klein MB. Patterns and outcomes of pediatric facial fractures in the United States: A survey of the National Trauma Data Bank. *J Am Coll Surg.* 2008 Nov;207(5):710–716. doi: 10.1016/j.jamcollsurg.2008.06.333. Epub 2008 Aug 9. Erratum in: *J Am Coll Surg.* 2009 Feb;208(2):325. PMID: 18954784; PMCID: PMC3049162.

5.   Smartt JM Jr, Low DW, Bartlett SP. The pediatric mandible: II. Management of traumatic injury or fracture. *Plast Reconstr Surg.* 2005 Aug;116(2):28e–41e. doi: 10.1097/01.prs.0000173445.10908.f8. PMID: 16079655.

6.   Lewis CJ, Robert LF,2.5 — Pediatric Mandible Fractures,Editor(s): Amir H. Dorafshar, Eduardo D. Rodriguez, Paul N. Manson, *Facial Trauma Surgery*, Elsevier, 2020, Pages 323–335, ISBN 9780323497558.

7.   Granick MS, Tran BNN, Alvarez OM. Latest advances in wound debridement techniques. *Surg Technol Int.* 2020 May 28;36:37–40. PMID: 32250443.

8.   Zimmermann CE, Troulis MJ, Kaban LB. Pediatric facial fractures: Recent advances in prevention, diagnosis and management. *Int J Oral Maxillofac Surg.* 2006 Jan;35(1):2–13. doi: 10.1016/j.ijom.2005.09.014. PMID: 16425444.

Chapter 6

Dentoalveolar Trauma

Mohammed Sumair Khan

Introduction

This chapter provides an outline of the management of dental trauma for clinicians with limited dental experience. Craniofacial injuries often involve dentition and may need to be treated by those without any dental experience. We aim to cover the recognition of dental care from treating a single painful tooth to the restoration of displaced teeth, with the aid of illustrative cases.

Key points for the non-specialist to be aware of:

- Check for loose fragments of tooth/bone/dentures which could choke the patient (Figure 6.1).
- Be aware that alveolar bone is different from other bones as it has a rich blood supply to aid the healing process and a high osteointegration rate. It is important not to discard it in the way that a surgeon might do with other damaged bones.
- Intraoral injuries require delicate manipulation of soft tissue, and it is important to cover any exposed alveolar bone with soft tissue. Due to the rich blood supply to the area, it is likely that there will be greater levels of bleeding but this can be controlled

by a pressure gauze with suction. Healing and osseointegration occur faster in this region.

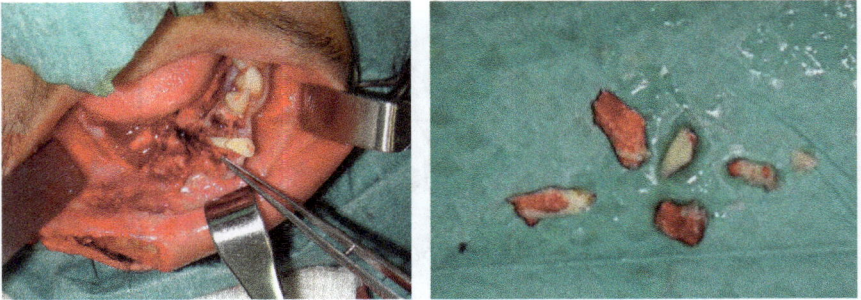

Figure 6.1   Blast injury causing loss of soft tissue (right-lower lip), damage to the dentoalveolar area of mandible, and fractured fragments of teeth and bone which are a choking hazard. Misrata war, 2011.

Orofacial Examination

Prior to treating patients with dental problems, it is important to take a full medical history where possible and consider any relevant disorders or regular medication.

It is essential to establish if oral pain is dental in origin due to inflammation or if it is a case of idiopathic odontalgia which can resemble common dental pain (see Chapter 7).

For this, a standard patient questionnaire is invaluable. However, in a war zone or other emergency situations, this may not be possible, and the clinician has to assess the patient's fitness quickly and concentrate on the emergency procedure. Also, it is likely that the patient will have already been assessed in the medical field hospital or clinic, so this would be repetitious.

The dental examination should include:

- an intraoral examination of the teeth, gingiva, oral mucosa, tongue, palate, and oropharynx;

- tooth vitality testing (discussed below);
- externally — the examination of the face, including the lips, lymph nodes of the neck, and palpation of the submandibular and parotid salivary glands. Also, check the temporomandibular joints (TMJ) and the dental occlusion, which may present with painful clicking and limited opening (trismus) (see Chapter 7). In children, it is important to be aware of the growth centres in the TMJ area.

It is often impossible to examine a patient with a maxillofacial injury at initial presentation, and they may need an anaesthetic or conscious sedation.

Tooth Vitality Testing

Vitality testing is an essential means of establishing the prognosis of a tooth by establishing a **diagnosis** of tooth vitality.

Currently there are two types of pulp test:

1. Sensitivity testing of the pulp by its response to hot, cold, and electric stimulus.
2. Vitality testing which assesses the blood supply within the tooth.

There are four possible outcomes of the pulp sensitivity test:

1. Normal response: A healthy pulp responds to sensitivity testing, which is a short, sharp pain which subsides when the stimulus is removed.
2. Heightened or prolonged lingering response: This indicates a degree of pulpal inflammation, which subsides once the stimulus has been removed.
3. Lingering pain: Continuing pain after the removal of the stimulus is indicative of irreversible pulpitis.
4. Nil response: This suggests that the nerve supply to the tooth is necrotic or has been root treated.

There are some limitations to sensitivity testing as heat tests may cause damage to the teeth and surrounding mucosa. Furthermore, the use of electric pulp testing has been questioned for patients with cardiac pacemakers despite the lack of evidence. Also, a tooth being tested adjacent to metallic restorations can create electrical conduction and yield false results.

Classifications of Traumatised Teeth

Traumatised teeth usually present with bleeding from the gingival margin which indicates a fracture of the underlying bone. There are two main methods of classification of the outcome of trauma.[1,2] The first considers the tooth as a whole and has the following categories:

Concussion

This is injury to the supporting structure of an intact tooth with no abnormal mobility or displacement. The tooth is tender to percussion and may also bleed from the gingivae.

Luxation Injuries

- Subluxation: This is injury to the supporting structure of a tooth with loosening but without displacement. The tooth is tender to percussion and bleeds from the gingivae.
- Extrusive luxation: This injury causes outward displacement of the teeth.
- Intrusive luxation: This injury causes inward displacement of the teeth.[3]

Avulsion

This is where one or more teeth are displaced from the socket but may be replanted (Figures 6.2–6.4).[4]

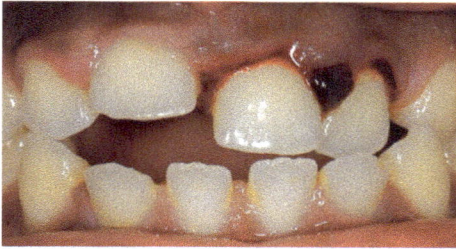

Figure 6.2 Luxation (anterior view): This patient was struck in the face and the upper-left central and lateral incisors were palatally displaced.

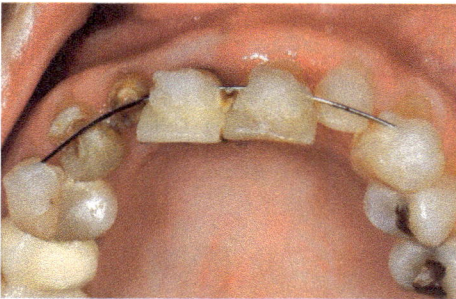

(a)

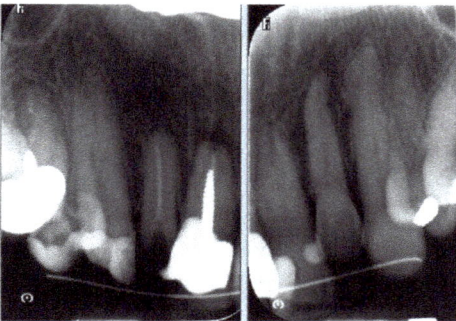

(b)

Figure 6.3 Luxation: *This patient suffered a blow which mobilised the upper central incisors;* (a) Upper central incisors were stabilised by being splinted to the first premolars with cement and wire. Upper-right lateral incisor and canine were carious and previously fractured; (b) Periapical radiographs taken one week after the acute trauma showed the upper-right central and lateral incisors survived despite being previously root filled. The central incisor was a crown replacement.

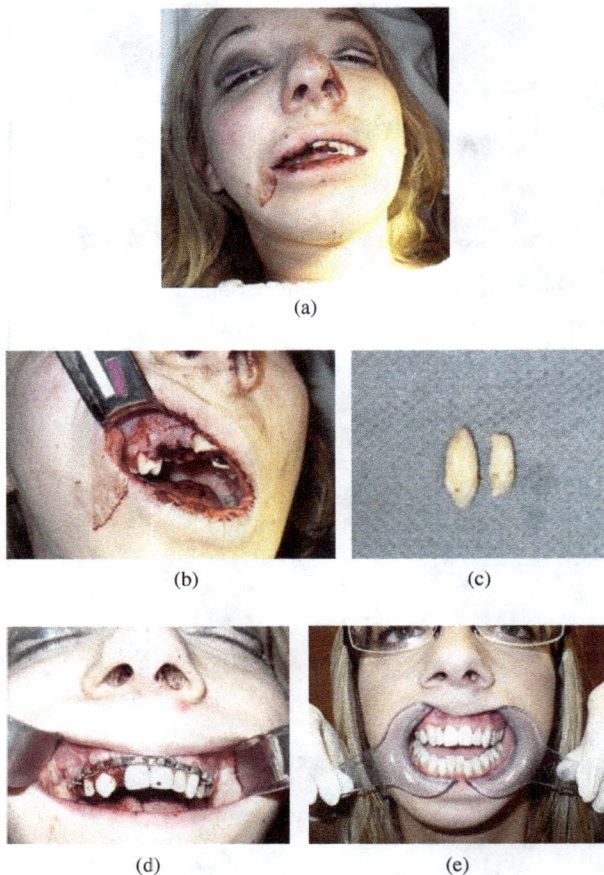

Figure 6.4   (a) A 24-year-old patient suffered right maxillary dentoalveolar trauma with two avulsed teeth. The upper-right canine was preserved with root canal therapy and a veneer to ensure its aesthetics, and the upper-right lateral incisor was replaced with a partial denture. Courtesy of Prof. Sabah Kalamchi; (b) and (c) Missing avulsed upper-right lateral incisor and canine; (d) Under local anaesthesia and intravenous sedation, the avulsed teeth were replanted and stabilised with an Erich arch bar; (e) Final replantation of the upper-right canine and replacement of the upper-right lateral incisor with a denture.

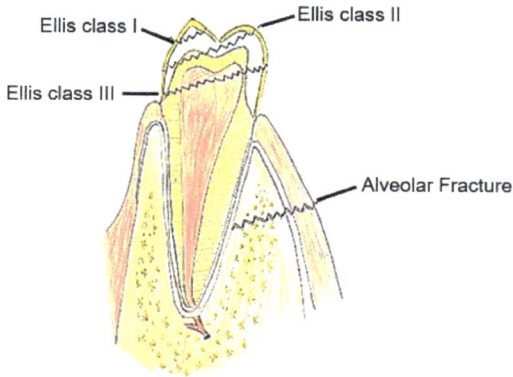

Figure 6.5   Fractured molar showing the three stages of a crown fracture: I, II, and III. (Ellis and Davey Classification, 1970).

Examples of Traumatised Teeth

A second, alternative classification of traumatised teeth is in terms of tooth structure. This is Ellis's classification of an undisplaced fractured crown (Figure 6.5):

Ellis Class I

The fracture is confined to the enamel. Treatment: Relieve any sharp margins and restore any defect where needed.

Ellis Class II

Enamel and dentine involvement. Treatment: Sensitivity reveals the vitality of the tooth. Protect the exposed dentine with a cement to restore the tooth.

Ellis Class III

'Complicated' fractures which involve the loss of the enamel and dentine with pulp exposure. Treatment: Provide pulp protection or a partial pulpotomy to protect the vitality with a lining cement. Cover with a temporary restoration or crown. Re-evaluate in four to six weeks to assess viability.

Root fractures may occur in severe trauma cases, where the coronal tissue remains intact and the fracture occurs in the root of the tooth below the gingival margin.

Examples of 'complicated' fractures (Figures 6.6–6.8):

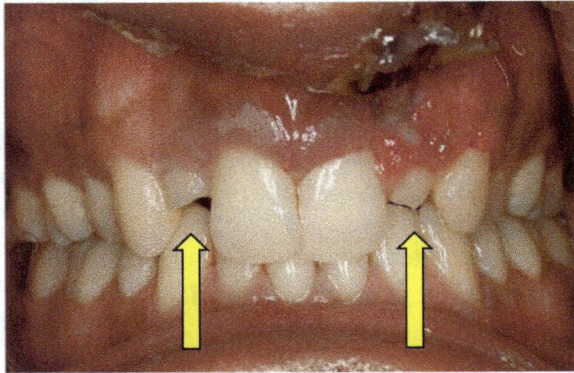

Figure 6.6 Coronal fractures of two upper lateral incisors with pulp exposure, caused by an assault.

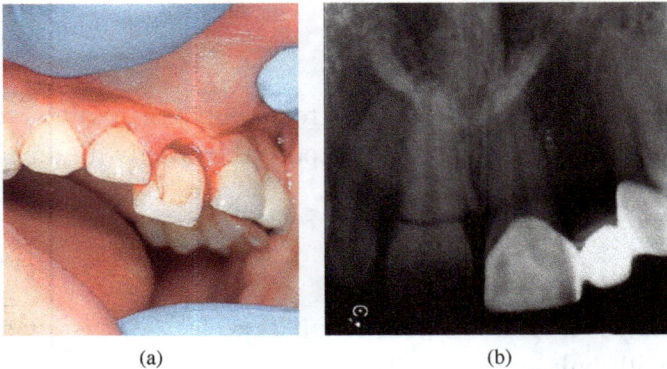

(a) (b)

Figure 6.7 (a) and (b) Horizontal root fracture of upper-right central incisor caused by a fist blow.

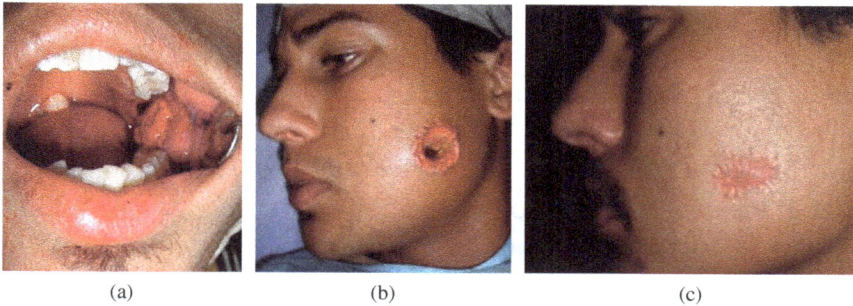

Figure 6.8　(a–c) Bullet-caused soft-tissue injury and fracture of the upper-left second molar (the fractured crown still posteriorly at the patient oral cavity). Misrata war, 2011.

Dental Radiographs

(Also see Chapter 7)

Although single periapical radiographs are invaluable for assessing individual teeth, a panoramic X-ray has greater value to investigate the following:

- fractures of the jaws;
- position of a crown fracture in relation to the dental pulp;
- stage of root development of a child;
- position of dislodged (luxated) teeth;
- peri-apical pathology;
- pathology of the temporo-mandibular joints;
- floor of the maxillary sinuses.

Treatment of Traumatised Teeth

Enamel and Dentine Fractures

These should be dealt with as an emergency measure to stop painful sensitivity of the exposed dentine. The dentine can be sealed with an adhesive material, such as a glass ionomer cement or composite resin.

The pulp vitality must be established prior to provision of any definitive restoration. If the pulp dies, then endodontic treatment is essential and should not be delayed.

A delay in providing root canal treatment can result in apical infection and discolouration of the tooth due to necrotic pulp products. If the dental pulp becomes necrotic and infected, a full pulpectomy is essential. This requires the removal of the pulp contents to be replaced by a root filling.

Symptoms of a pulp infection include pain caused by hot or cold food and drink as well as pain during biting or chewing. These symptoms disappear as the pulp dies, until a dental abscess arises with a painful facial swelling. Antibiotics alone are ineffective in treating root canal infections which require removal under a local anaesthetic.

If neglected, this can develop into a serious infection in the facial spaces (Figure 6.9). In severe cases, this could develop into Ludwig's Angina (as described in Chapter 4) and become life threating.

A non-infected partial pulp treatment, called a 'partial Cvek pulpotomy', prevents pain and microbial invasion. Clinical and radiographic follow up is usually after two weeks and then at four-week intervals, three further times.

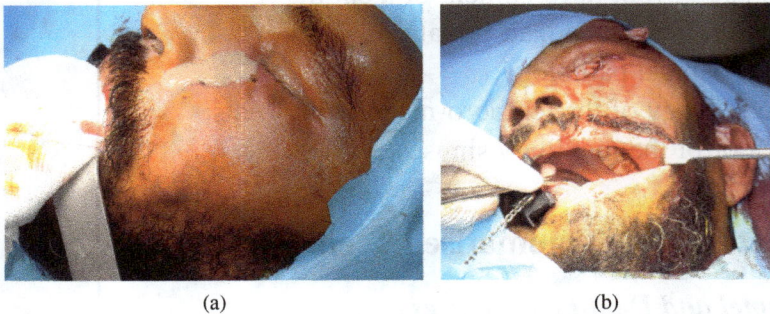

(a)   (b)

Figure 6.9   (a) and (b) Neglected dental infection of the upper-left teeth. The dental abscess spread in the left facial space including the orbital area (orbital cellulitis). It was treated under General Anaesthetics (GA) by incision and drainage (intraoral, infraorbital supraorbital, and preauricular drain), extraction of infected teeth, and antibiotics.

Periodontal Status

Healthy alveolar bone is essential to provide sound support for the teeth which are suspended by the 'fibre ligaments' of the periodontal membrane and the overlying gingivae. If neglected, the teeth may develop a biofilm plaque of microorganisms that accumulates on the tooth surface and cause inflamed gingivae which bleed and induce caries, periodontitis, and abscess formation.

Once dental restorations have been provided, oral hygiene procedures should be established, including tooth brushing and interproximal cleansing aids, such as dental floss. The lamina dura is a compact bone lining the tooth socket. The lamina dura provides the attachment of Sharpey's fibres of the periodontal ligament. On an X-ray, the lamina dura will appear as a fine radiopaque line surrounding the tooth root. Assessment of the lamina dura will help define the periodontal status regarding infections.

Bone Grafting

Violence can predispose to dental trauma with bone loss requiring a graft.

In the past, dentoalveolar trauma would not attract attention, but recent advances in dental treatment including dental implants include a variety of techniques to preserve the natural dentoalveolar structure.

Example of Bone Grafting

This patient suffered premaxillary trauma and extractions leaving a bone defect from the upper-right lateral incisor to the upper-left second premolar which required a graft (Figure 6.10).

During the stabilisation phase, the patient was provided with a partial acrylic denture. The upper-left lateral incisor was restored with a composite resin restoration and kept out of occlusion while its vitality was monitored. The definitive treatment phase took six months after bone grafting.

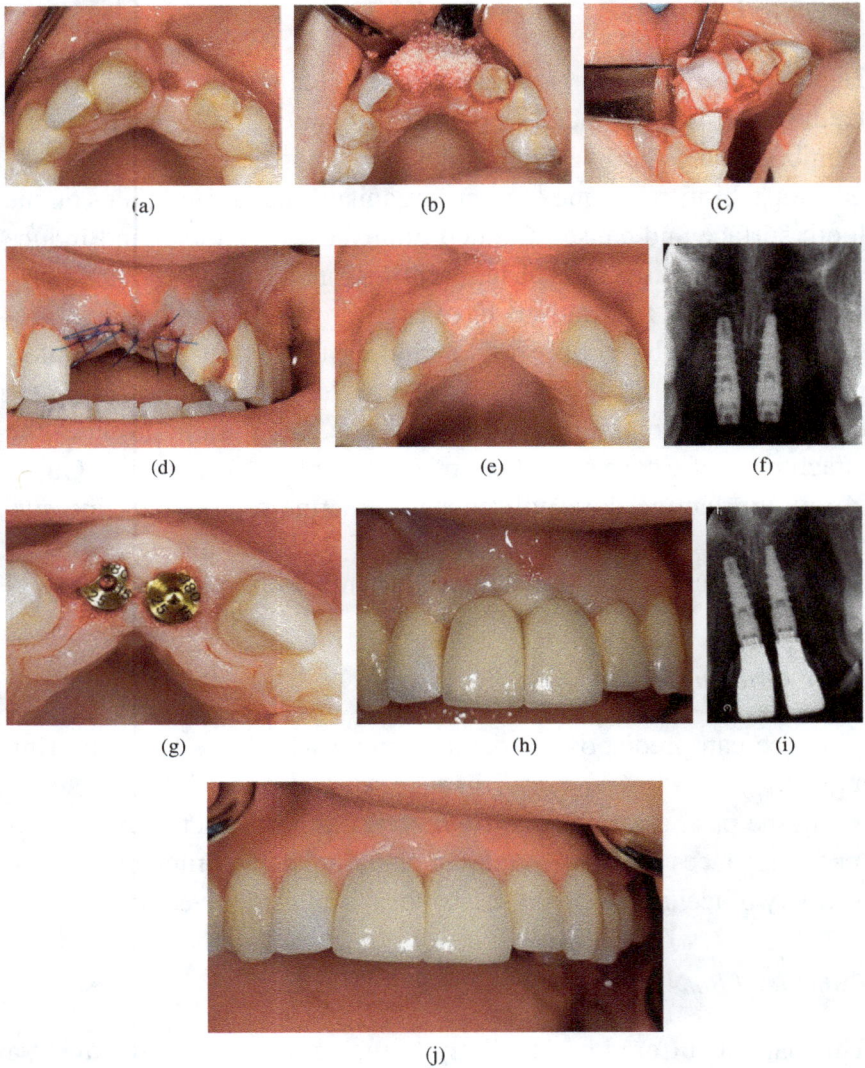

Figure 6.10   (a) Initial presentation; (b) Dentoalveolar extraction defects were grafted with a mixture of autogenous and bovine particulate bone; (c) Graft was covered with a collagen membrane; (d) Mucosal flap closure was achieved with prolene sutures; (e) Dental implants were placed in the upper-left and -right central incisor positions; (f) CT scan of implant placement; (g) Implants uncovered; (h) and (i) Implants and definitive crowns fitted; (j) Post-implant review.

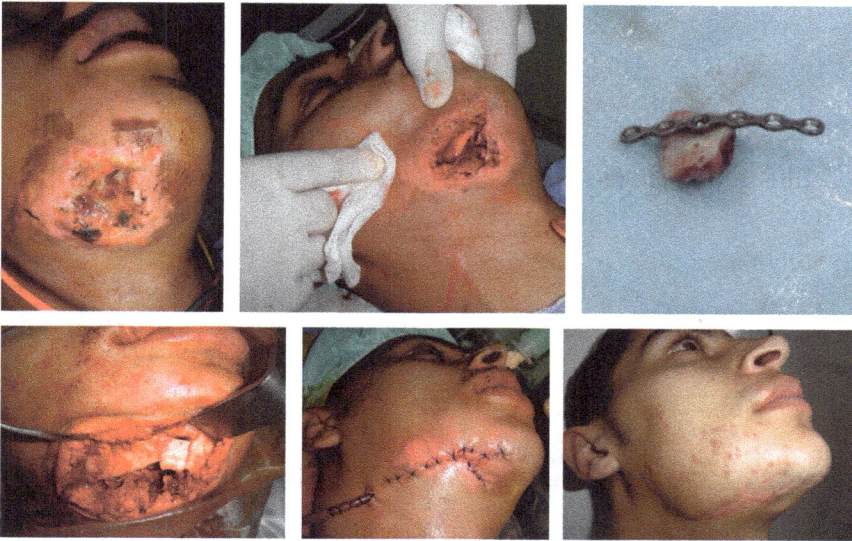

Figure 6.11   Successfully re-using a bone fragment.

In war trauma, it is better wherever possible to keep bone fragments in their original position, fixed with stainless-steel wire or screws. This will preserve the jaw's continuity, avoid bone grafting, and facilitate rehabilitation in the future (Figure 6.11).

Aftercare

After the initial emergency treatment, follow up and aftercare are likely to be performed by a dental specialist:

- After severe trauma with the loss of teeth and alveolar bone, the support for the lips may need to be restored.
- Following the stabilisation phase, the final position of the missing teeth can be established with a temporary denture or bridge.
- The periodontal status must be stable and maintained with an ideal level of oral hygiene. Oral hygiene neglect may lead to

serious circumstances, such as pain, spread of infection, and loss of teeth. Only then should the patient be offered fixed prostheses for any missing teeth.

Illustrative Cases of Dental War Injuries (Figures 6.12 and 6.13):

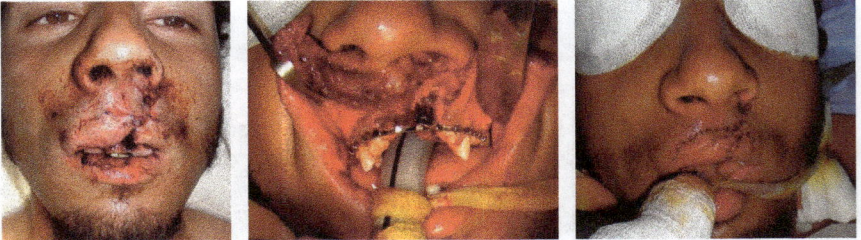

Figure 6.12   Blast-injury-caused soft-tissue injury and fracture of alveolar bone and upper anterior teeth, (under GA, soft-tissue management, alveolar bone fixation used arch bar). Misrata war, 2011.

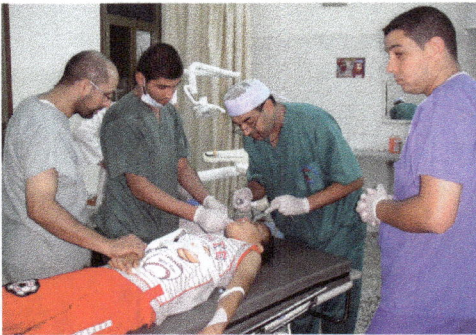

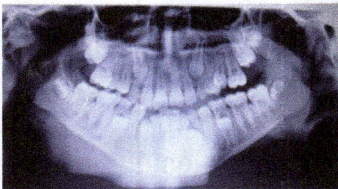

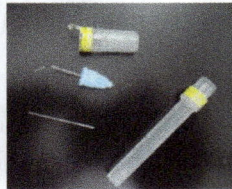

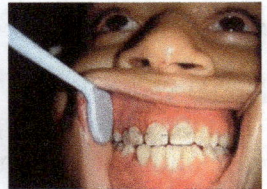

Figure 6.13   An 11-year-old boy sustained blunt trauma which caused a greenstick mandibular fracture to the right (treated conservatively), upper-right teeth displacement fixed with stainless-steel wire and composite. Misrata war, 2011.

References

1. Berman LH, Blanco L, Cohen S. *A Clinical Guide to Dental Traumatology* (China, Mosby Elsevier, 2007).
2. Bimstein E, Rotstein I. Cvek pulpotomy — revisited. *Dent Traumatol.* 2016 Jul;32(6):438–442. doi: 10.1111/edt.12297.
3. Bourguignon C, Cohhenca N, Lauridsen E, Flores MT, O'Connell AC, Day PF, Tsilingardis G, Abbot PV, Fouad AF, Hicks L, Andreasen JO, Cehreli ZC, Harlamb S, Kahler B, Oginni A, Spencer M, Levin L. International association of dental traumatology guidelines for the management of traumatic dental injuries: 1. Fractures and luxations. *Dent Traumatol.* 2020 May;36(4):314–330.
4. Fouad AF, Abbot PV, Tsilingardis G, Cohenca N, Lauridsen E, Bourguignon C, O'Connell AC, Flores MT, Day PF, Hicks L, Andreasen JO, Cehreli ZC, Harlamb S, Kahler B, Oginni A, Semper M, Levin L. International association of dental traumatology guidelines for the management of traumatic dental injuries: 2. Avulsion of permanent teeth. *Dent Traumatol.* 2020 May;36(4):331–342.

Chapter 7

Craniofacial Imaging

Malcolm Harris and Abdulhakim Zaggut

Introduction

Battlefield radiology is like any other field of radiology in that it requires specific knowledge of aetiology (mechanism of injury), common patterns of disease (injury patterns), and the same list of presentations to search for in a patient radiograph. Advanced scanners (computed tomography (CT), magnetic resonance imaging (MRI)) require training before being operated by radiologists and radiographers; however, this chapter focuses on imaging techniques commonly used in war zones specifically for craniofacial injuries.

Radiographs of the facial skeleton and dentition are an essential step in the management ladder, integrating imaging and overall patient management. The management of facial gunshot wounds and blast injuries follows the advanced trauma life support (ATLS) regime (see Chapter 2).

In ideal circumstances, imaging should include a CT scan with 3-D reconstruction to exclude complex facial fractures and a panoramic radiograph mainly for alveolar bone and dentation, but if these are not available, basic head and neck X-rays can be useful.

The plain X-ray is an important element in managing war casualties as a rapid method to detect potential threats to the airway, including laryngeal injury, aspirated teeth, and intraoral swelling as well as cervical spine fractures.

After the patient passes the emergency stage and stabilises, a thorough examination is required, including radiological imaging to detect complex craniofacial fractures to plan for further treatment for example, detection of malocclusion to exclude fractures of the mandible, maxilla, and zygomas.

Many publications discuss current war surgery from well-equipped military battlefield hospitals with deployed doctors and staff who have been trained for such environments. Furthermore, these hospitals are well-equipped and generally located in safe areas, thus allowing staff to perform, with less likelihood of encountering fighting. In contrast, a civilian war zone scene is vastly different with a lack of specialist surgeons and limited medical supplies and equipment, particularly radiology machines. Even if available, there can be power cuts or insufficient electricity generated for large CT scanners; therefore, a return to basic and classical techniques in treating casualties become essential in such environments.

History

While studying the effects of passing an electrical current through gases at low pressure, the German physicist, Wilhelm Rontgen, inadvertently discovered X-rays (Figure 7.1). X-ray is an electromagnetic, high-energy, and ionising radiation.

Within a year, the first radiology department opened in a Glasgow hospital and produced pictures of a renal calculus and a penny lodged in a child's throat. During the Greco–Turkish War of 1897, X-rays were used for diagnostic purposes for the first time near a battlefield in a mobile military vehicle. This was a major

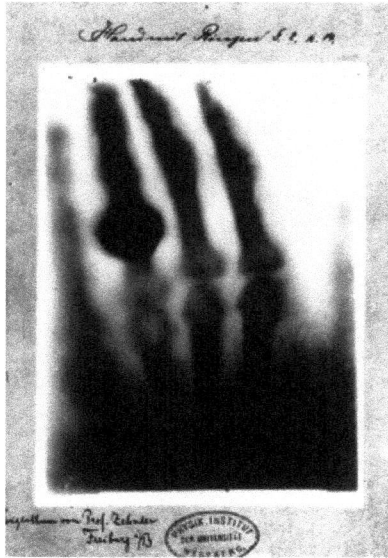

Figure 7.1   The first X-ray of Rontgen's wife's hand (1895).

development towards the creation of the motor-ambulance service. During World War I, the Polish physicist and chemist, Marie Curie, trained radiologists and developed mobile X-ray cars to work at the front line[1] (Figure 7.2).

Her research introduced the major development of radiographs into surgery, and she later became the head of the radiological services for the International Red Cross, also organising training courses for medical staff in new diagnostic techniques. Marie Curie dedicated her work to improving healthcare in field hospitals but died from leukaemia due to excessive exposure to high-energy radiation from her research.[1,2] X-ray images were the first type of medical imaging used by doctors; however, as X-ray radiation is able to penetrate human tissue and bone, it has been linked to side effects ranging from vomiting and hair loss to cancer. X-ray machines at the time were not designed to scan the face and skull,

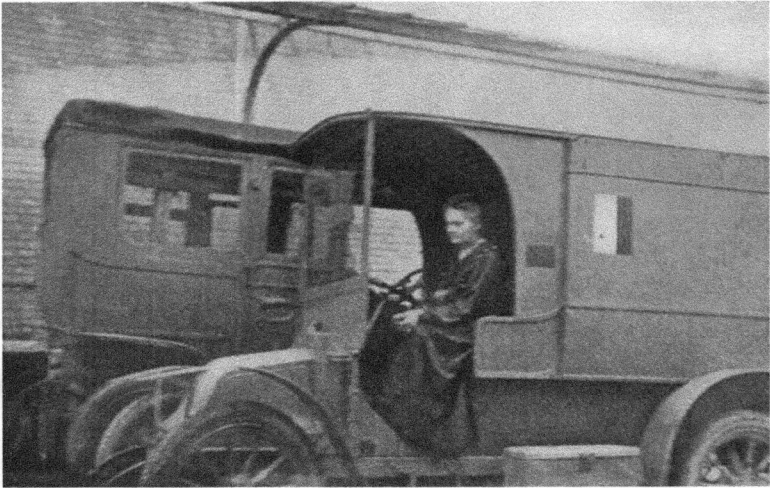

Figure 7.2   Marie Curie in one of the original mobile radiology units that she devised for use in war, ca. 1915.

resulting in dental and medical specialists collaboratively developing X-ray machines for the face (Figure 7.3).[2]

Imaging of Craniofacial Fractures

The availability of images of craniofacial fractures depends on the facilities available in war and austere environments. Various types of radiographs can be used to help confirm diagnosis and identify fractures.

Dental and Direct Digital Radiograph

For the management of primary trauma, the presence of direct digital radiograph (DDR) fixed or portable X-ray machines are essential in emergency rooms. DDR is used to display fractures in high resolution as high doses of X-ray are used. Although this is a reliable and fast method for imaging, it is not a preferred imaging method

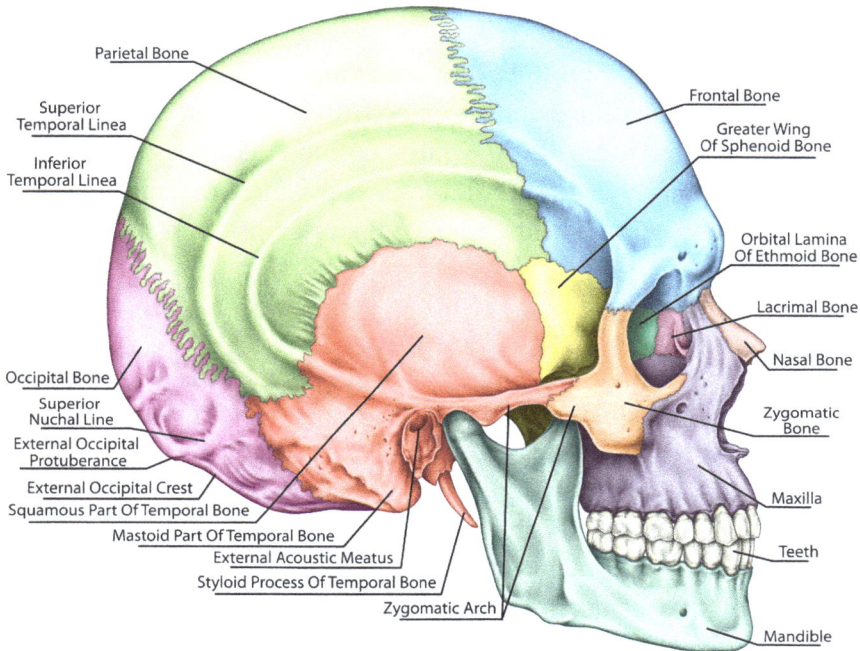

Figure 7.3   Skull and facial bones.

due to high radiation exposure but invaluable for surgeons in war zones. Surgeons commonly request multiple images of the craniofacial area, taken at 90° intervals:

- **Occipitomental (OM) view:** OM0° shows facial bones and maxillary sinus and is helpful in the assessment of midface, orbit, and zygoma fractures. OM30° is useful for showing mandibular coronoid process and same as OM0°.
- **Posteroanterior (PA) view:** This shows mandibular lower border and mandibular condyle.
- **Lateral view:** This shows posterior mandible.
- **Anteroposterior (AP) view:** This is used for cervical spine imaging.

Panoramic Radiographs

The orthopantomograph (OPG) is a panoramic radiograph that produces a two-dimensional image of both the upper and lower jaws, spanning from ear to ear. It is the most common radiograph in oral and maxillofacial surgery and helpful for the assessment of teeth, alveolar, and jawbone (Figure 7.4). Its value is discussed in Chapter 6.

Dental Radiographs

(1) Periapical radiograph (Figure 7.5) shows the full length of the tooth and the surrounding alveolar bone, helpful to detect fractures and abnormalities.
(2) Occlusal radiograph (Figures 7.6(a) and (b)) provides a broader field of view and can show either upper or lower occlusal view of dental and alveolar bone, lower anterior mandibular fractures, nasopalatine canal, impacted teeth, nasomaxillary cyst, and a stone of submandibular duct (anterior part).

Computed Tomography

CT scans use several X-ray images and computer processing to create cross-sectional images (Figure 7.7). In case of an emergency, such as

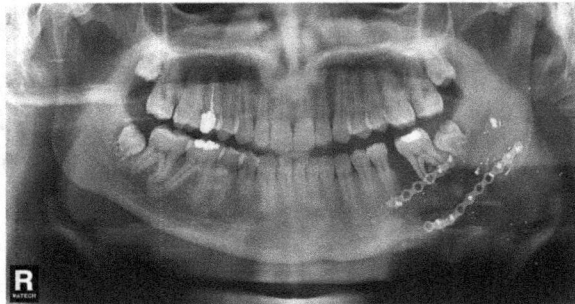

Figure 7.4 A blast injury: panoramic radiograph showing a fracture of the left side of the mandible which was treated with mini-plates and screws.

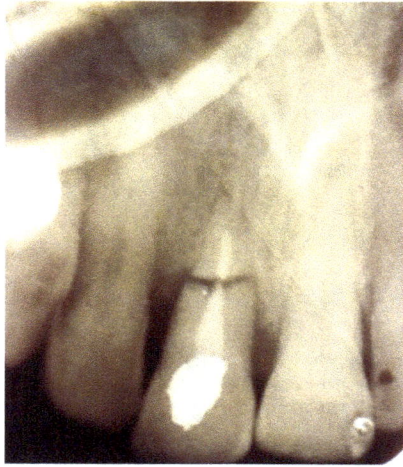

Figure 7.5   Periapical radiograph showing a fractured central incisor root and periapical radiolucency.

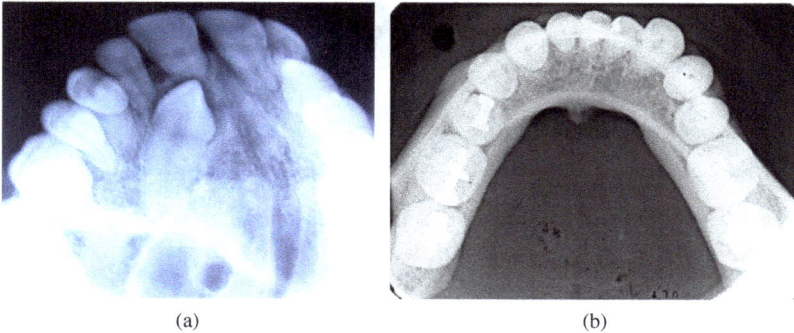

(a)   (b)

Figure 7.6   (a) Occlusal view of impacted canine and incisive foramen; (b) Occlusal radiograph of a normal mandible.

airway crisis or uncontrolled bleeding, a patient would not benefit from a CT scanner which provides very high-resolution images.

CT scans have various usages in the trauma field; they are useful for head and neck scan in severe Craniomaxillofacial (CMF) trauma cases as a large amount of information can be obtained before surgery or treatment takes place. CT scanner staff are required to

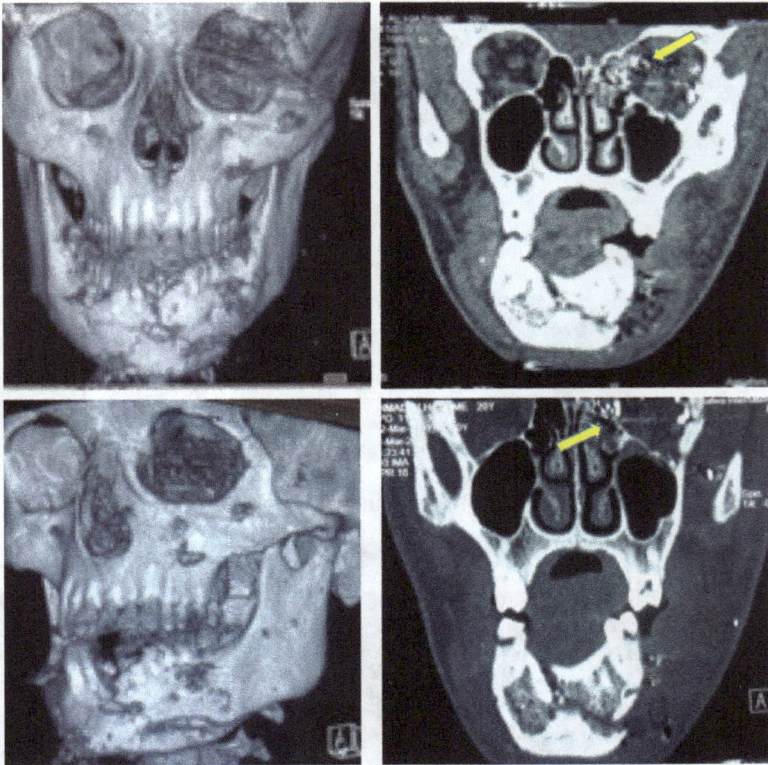

Figure 7.7   CT scan of blast injury producing comminuted splintered mandible, left ethmoid injury, and perforation of left orbit (arrow).

prepare the machine beforehand as scans cannot be taken at such short notice. Given access to a CT scanner in an emergency situation, brain scans are taken first followed by the facial bone. In the case of war injuries, it is more useful for the surgeon to fully utilise the three-dimensional (3-D) modelling capabilities of the machine. This provides the surgeons a detailed 3-D reconstruction of fractures and damages, which is particularly useful for orbital and midface trauma. In the case of aesthetic surgeries, CT scans provide very detailed images. CT scans can also be used for finding the source of cerebrospinal fluid (CSF) leaks, skull defects, craniofacial deformities, and angiograms.

Cone Beam Computed Tomography (CBCT)

CBCT is a more advanced form of CT imaging that exposes the patient to less radiation than conventional CT, is more affordable, and shows finer details such as inferior alveolar nerve, Temporomandibular joint (TMJ) pathology, fractures of zygomatic bone, complex, orbital, condyle, and neck (Figure 7.8).

Sialography

This is the specific examination of salivary glands involving the injection of a contrast dye into the salivary duct. An X-ray is performed allowing for the assessment of dilatations and strictures. Stones can be detected in salivary glands by injection into the canula to gland duct.

Magnetic Resonance Imaging

MRI uses strong magnetic fields and radio waves to create diagnostic images which are precise details of body parts, especially of soft

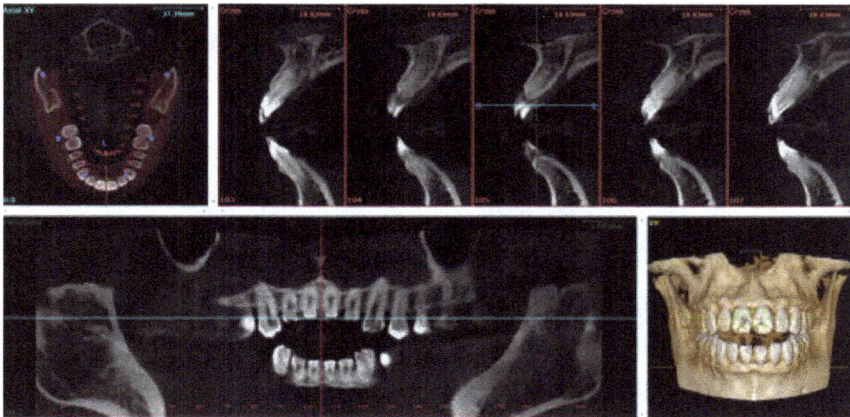

Figure 7.8   CBCT image.
Source: Image licensed under CC BY-SA 4.0. By Panda 51.

tissues (Figure 7.10). MRI scanners do not cause any physiological damage but cannot be used with patients with metal implants, such as cochlea implants or pacemakers. MRI scans provide good-quality images of intraoral soft tissue, brain tissue, salivary glands, tongue, and TMJ disc, which can be combined with intravenous contrast and are useful for vascular and osteomyelitis assessments. MRI scanners are particularly large and expensive; therefore, their availability is limited in austere environments. There are various MRI-based imaging techniques (Figures 7.9 and 7.10):

- **Functional MRI (fMRI)** measures blood flow to assess brain activity.
- **Nuclear magnetic resonance (NMR)** spectroscopy is the study of molecules by recording the interaction of radiofrequency electromagnetic radiations with the nuclei of molecules placed in a strong magnetic field. It is commonly used for brain scans.
- **Positron emission tomography (PET)** uses radiotracers to assess organ and tissue functions. For concussion, it is used to

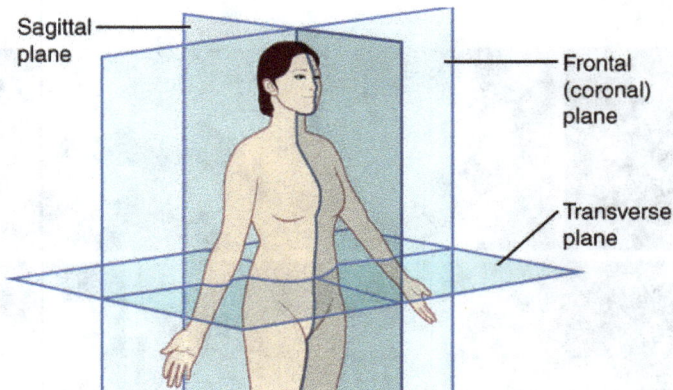

Figure 7.9   CT and MRI scanning requires familiarity with imaging planes.

Source: Image licensed under CC BY-SA 3.0. By Connexions, OpenStax College, Anatomy & Physiology, Connexions Website. http://cnx.org/content/col11496/1.6/, June 19, 2013.

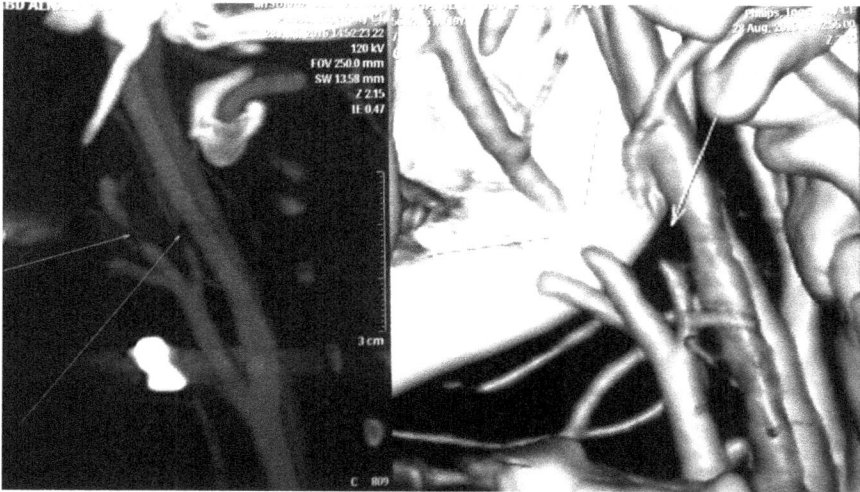

Figure 7.10 MRI scan showing the relation of shrapnel to the blood vessels in the neck.

study the development of abnormal tau tangles. These neurofibrillary tangles are insoluble twisted fibres found inside the brain cells and are known to be a feature of chronic trauma.

- **Nuclear Imaging** is used in with combination with CT scans for higher-resolution images. Although an expensive option, this can be used to assess recurrent and metastases of tumours of the brain as well as the base of the tongue.

Ultrasonography

Ultrasound is non-invasive and utilises sound waves with frequencies higher than the upper audible limit of human hearing. As the sound waves travel through your body, the pattern of refraction can be interpreted by computers to produce an image. This method is useful for soft-tissue imaging, such as salivary glands, neck lumps, cystic lesions, blood, and pus collections.

Examples of Craniofacial Radiography

To this day, a basic radiograph is an invaluable and immediate diagnostic tool for clinicians on the front line. More treatment may be required for facial fractures in both adults and children with further radiographic and computerised imaging.

In war zones, primary management includes the control of intracranial and facial bleeding as well as detection of fractures of the cervical spine. The bleeding skull base may also be manifested by a subcutaneous mastoid ecchymosis (Battle's sign). With the development of radiographic techniques, attention can be focused on the facial skeleton and dentoalveolar structures.

Mandibular Fractures

Mandible fractures are among the most frequently seen injuries in the trauma centre setting.[3]

Radiological Views of the Fractured Mandible

In austere environments and war zones, the most common X-ray view available is the plain X-ray which can provide useful information in a short space of time (Figure 7.11).

Maxillofacial Fractures and Le Fort Classification

Classification of Maxillary Fractures

Medical literature commencing from the early 20th century has developed several classification systems to serve different purposes. Rene Le Fort (1869–1951) introduced the first midface fracture classification which became known as Le Fort I, II, and III based on the fracture pattern of facial bones obtained by boiling the soft tissue to separate the fractured bones when examining crush injuries in cadavers (Figures 7.12 and 7.13).

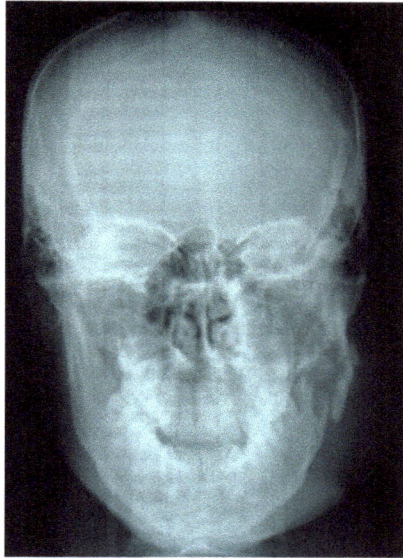

Figure 7.11   Frontal (Postero-anterior) X-ray showing a mandibular fracture of the left mandible angle.

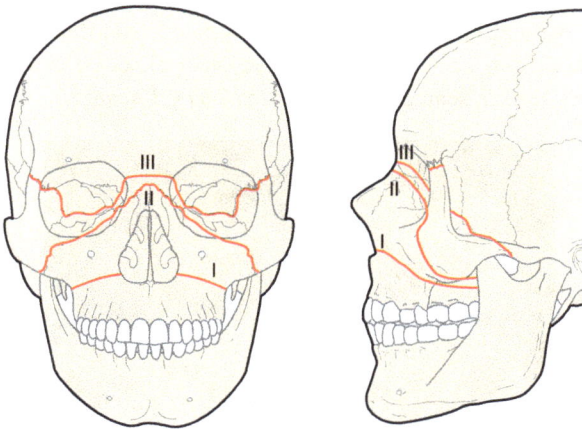

Figure 7.12   Le Fort classification of maxillary fractures.

Zygomatic Fractures

The zygoma or malar bone represents the prominence of the cheek above, lateral to, and below the orbit. The zygoma articulates with

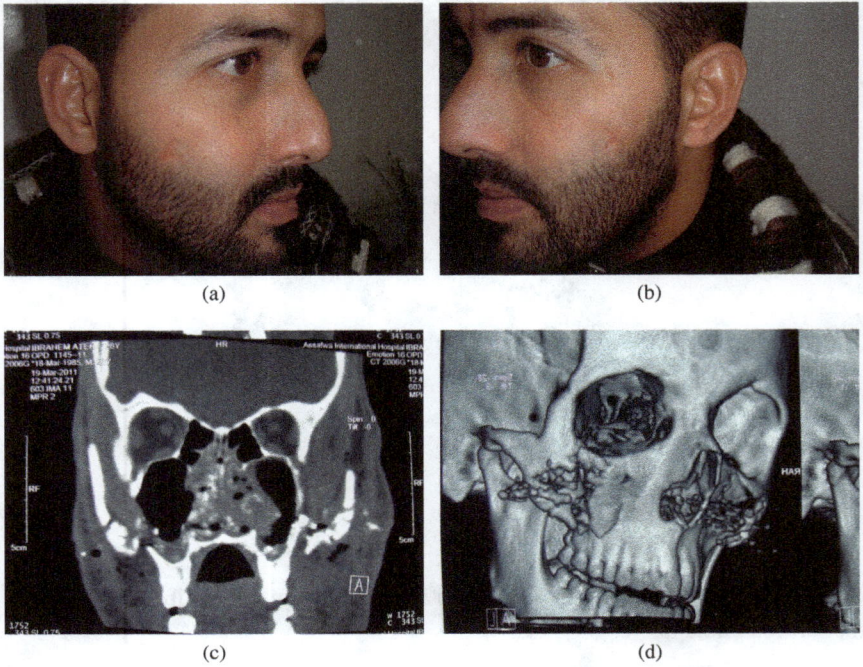

(a)

(b)

(c)

(d)

Figure 7.13   (a) and (b) Le Fort I fracture caused by a bullet which passed through the face from one side and out the other (known as a 'through-and-through' injury); (c) CT scan corona view; (d) 3-D CT scan.

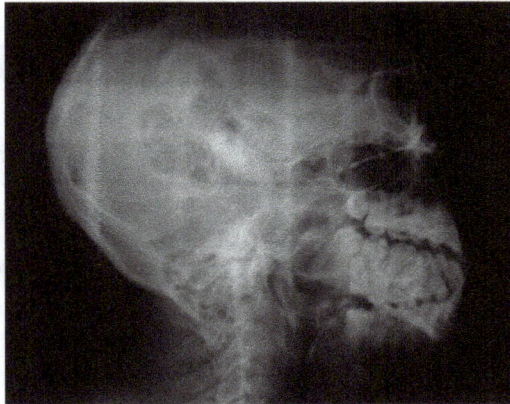

Figure 7.14   Example of a radiological view of a midface fracture.

the frontal bone above and provides the lateral wall of the orbit, along with the maxilla below and the sphenoid within the orbit (Figure 7.15).

Conclusion

Medical imaging techniques have developed over time in a number of aspects. The primary concern is the adverse effects of using high-frequency radiation on patients, thus magnetic resonance, ultra-sound, and radio-wave-based imaging have been developed. Imaging has become fast and efficient, reducing the amount of radiation that the patient is exposed to. Furthermore, the entire body can be scanned and rendered in interactive 3-D models providing detailed information. Additionally, fluorescent biomarkers can be ingested or injected and tracked in real time.

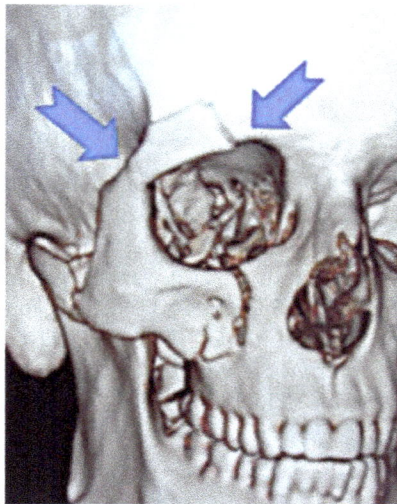

Figure 7.15   CT scan of a fractured zygoma.

With the advancement of technology and the desire to obtain the greatest levels of resolution, equipment in some cases has become more portable; however, it is not currently possible to reduce the size of an MRI machine. Furthermore, these machines require powerful computers to produce 3-D models. As a result, the power requirements are greater and often not sustainable in austere environments. So as the safer and more advanced imaging devices may not be available, X-rays are commonly used in war zones.

Despite the risks of X-ray exposure, it remains the cheapest, fastest, and most reliable imaging method. The main purpose of radiographic images and the plain-film X-rays is to identify hazards in the airway and determine the exact location and extension of craniofacial fractures and hazards adjacent to vital anatomical structures in order to determine if treatment is to be conservative or surgical. Radiology teams are vital in war surgery management because X-ray machines are easy to operate, the results are obtained quickly, and the results can be easily interpreted by surgeons. As a result, the use and interpretation of X-rays remains a vital skill in war zones.

References

1. Timothy J, Jorgensen TJ. How Marie Curie brought X-ray machines to the battlefield. 7 Dec 2018. https://www.smithsonianmag.com/history/how-marie-curie-brought-X-ray-machines-to-battlefield-180965240/.
2. Barclay A. Radiology in the first world war – Everything rad. 13 Nov 2014. https://www.carestream.com/blog/2014/11/13/radiology-first-world-war/.
3. Assael LA, Prein J. *Stable Internal Fixation of Osteotomies of the Facial Skeleton. Manual of Internal Fixation in the Cranio-Facial Skeleton* (Berlin, Germany, Springer Berlin Heidelberg, 1998), pp. 185–198.

Chapter 8

War Wound Management

Malcolm Harris

Introduction

Combat head and neck wounds are complex, especially when contaminated by debris from explosives. This complexity produces facial lacerations, fractured facial bones, and head injuries.

War wound care has evolved with modern technology; with digital imaging and telemedicine, combat wound images can be transmitted in advance to the hospital, while the patient is in transit.

Soft-tissue management of craniofacial patients requires a thorough medical history to exclude diabetes, smoking, alcohol, or radiation therapy, each of which inhibits wound healing. Also, an immunisation history may be important, in particular, for tetanus or rabies prophylaxis. In a war situation it is rarely possible to take this history in such detail and surgeons have to work with the information available.

Anatomy of the Skin

(1) **Epidermis:** This has five layers: stratum corneum, stratum lucidium, stratum granulosum, stratum spinosum, and stratum basale. Together, they comprise a waterproof barrier approximately 1.5 mm thick.

(2) **Dermis:** This is the connective tissue layer below the epidermis, which contains hair follicles, nerves, sweat glands, capillaries, and arterioles.

(3) **Hypodermis:** This contains fat, connective tissues, and blood vessels.

The anatomy of the skin is clearly shown in Figure 8.1.

Overview of Wound Management

- The choice of local or general anaesthesia will be determined by the severity of the wound and the state of the patient.

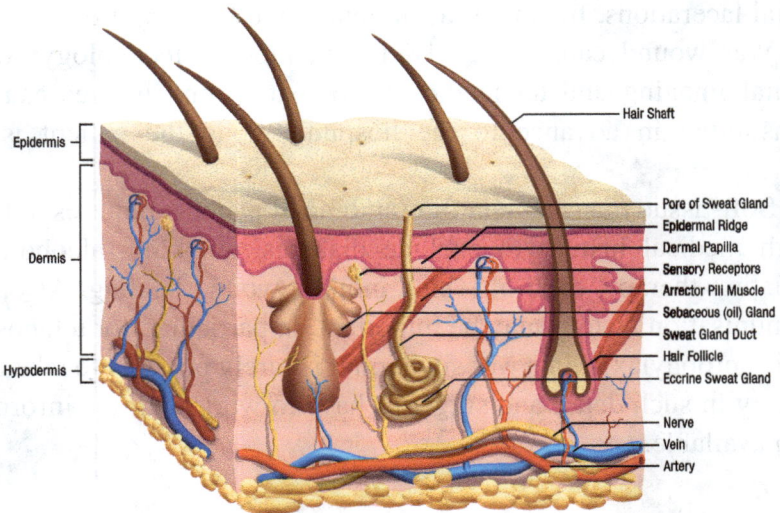

Figure 8.1   Anatomy of the skin.

- The patient is checked to identify all lesions, and in the case of a gunshot wound, both entry and exit wounds are examined. The most severe wounds are attended to first.
- Bleeding is arrested by applying pressure or surgical diathermy depending on the site and size of the wound.
- The surrounding area is debrided and cleansed. Note that there is no difference in infection rates in wounds cleansed with potable tap water compared with those cleaned with sterile normal saline.[1] However, it is appropriate to use sterile solutions for patients with compromised immunity, such as diabetic wounds, or where bone is exposed. The optimum temperature of any wound-cleansing solution should be 37°C i.e. body temperature. A colder solution impairs wound healing as a reduced wound temperature lowers oxygen levels and leucocyte counts.
- The wound size should be recorded by measuring the longest and broadest dimensions and the depth. The state of the underlying bone must also be recorded.
- The wound is dried and sutured. Alternatively, Steri-Strips are narrow adhesive bandages that are better than traditional sutures for limited wounds.
- The wound is dressed. Note that repeated removal and application of dressings can cause damage to the skin and predispose to infection.
- The patient is advised on follow-up analgesia.

Anaesthesia

Local anaesthesia is reliable and inexpensive where pain reduction is key to optimising the patient outcome. Even in a situation with limited resources, it enables prompt treatment with simple procedures, which will reduce the need for further surgery in the future.

Where possible, the clinician should use local anaesthesia to assess the injury and only consider general anaesthetic if local anaesthesia is ineffective.

The patient is informed that the local anaesthesia will block nerve conduction and control sharp pain but that the ability to feel some sensation of pressure will still remain.

Due to the rich blood supply in this region, anaesthetic agents are short-acting, but their duration can be lengthened by combining local anaesthesia with adrenaline.

An understanding of facial anatomy is essential for safe and effective local anaesthesia, and Chapter 4 contains detailed descriptions of how it should be administered (also see Chapter 2 for a discussion of general anaesthesia).

Antimicrobial Agents

Antibiotics

Antibiotics should not be administered for non-infected lesions or to patients with known allergies.

The selection of an antibiotic should be based on the culture and sensitivity of a swab if practicable. The appropriate choice can be from the following:

- Penicillin, amoxicillin, and co-amoxiclav (amoxicillin with anti-staphylococcus clavulanic acid);
- Erythromycin and clarithromycin are alternatives for penicillin allergy or penicillin-resistant strains of bacteria;
- Cephalosporins, such as cephalexin, for cases of septicaemia and meningitis;
- Aminoglycosides, such as gentamicin and tobramycin, for treatment of septicaemia;
- Anti-anaerobic antibiotics, including metronidazole and clindamycin.

Disinfectants

- Disinfectants are only used to eradicate microbes on dressing trolleys and surgical instruments. They are too aggressive to be used on a wound.

Antiseptics

Antiseptics are used to eradicate bacteria in a wound or on the intact skin of a pre-operative surgical site. They are also used for cleansing wounds with excessive exudate, necrotic tissue, or a biofilm. Antiseptics reduce the need for systemic antibiotics and avoid drug resistance.

After five days of using topical antiseptic solutions, the wound is re-assessed for signs of improvement which are reductions in slough or odour. If the wound has deteriorated or shows signs of a spreading infection, then systemic antibiotics are required.

Managing Biofilms

Bacteria are able to form complex surface-attached communities known as biofilms. They are 10 times more likely to form in chronic wounds than in acute ones, also preventing wound healing. The signs that a biofilm is involved are that the wound does not respond to treatment and persistent slough returns after debridement. Chronic wounds can be colonised by bacteria encased within a polymicrobial biofilm which produces a prolonged inflammatory response in the host. Polymicrobial biofilms also promote antibiotic resistance by allowing the transfer of antibiotic resistance genes.

Frequent debridement combined with the use of an antiseptic cleansing solution should be adequate for effective management.

Choice of Antiseptic

Antiseptics are available as irrigation solutions or gels and can be applied directly from the container onto a moistened wound or can be applied with a soaked gauze pad. This needs to be done at least once a day, and the gauze pad needs to be left on the wound for at least 15 minutes. Choices of antiseptics are as follows:

- **Polyhexanide and betaine (PHMB)** is less damaging to healthy cells than chlorhexidine and povidone iodine. A solution of 0.01–0.20% PHMB is recommended for heavily infected wounds with a contact time of 15 minutes.
- **Octenidine dihydrochloride** is active against Gram-positive and Gram-negative bacteria. This water-based solution is generally prescribed pre-operatively for the eradication of methicillin-resistant staphylococcus aureus and has broad-spectrum properties. It is effective for debriding slough and maintaining a moist environment, both of which help to disrupt biofilms in the wound bed. Octenidine dihydrochloride is not effective against viruses and spores.
- A **povidone–iodine fabric dressing** is a knitted viscose dressing with povidone–iodine incorporated in a hydrophilic polyethylene glycol base. The iodine has a wide spectrum of antimicrobial activity but is rapidly deactivated by wound exudate. The dressings are used as a wound contact layer for abrasions and superficial burns.
- **Manuka honey dressings** are used for shallow infected wounds. They have anti-bacterial, antioxidant, and anti-inflammatory properties.

Suturing Facial Lacerations

To avoid scars and a VII N (7th cranial nerve) palsy, when suturing a laceration to repair the nerve, care should be taken to recognise the branches of the VII N (see Fig. 4.5 of the facial nerve). A facial laceration involving the VII N can be repaired up to 24–48 h post injury, although six hours is the usual time for a contaminated wound. 4/0 nylon is the suture of choice. Absorbable sutures such as polyglycolic acid (3/0 or 4/0) can be used for intraoral mucosal lacerations e.g. when the patient will not return for suture removal or in a child for whom suture removal is difficult.

Interrupted sutures on the face should be placed close together for a cosmetically pleasing result, 1–2 mm from the skin edge and 3 mm apart to achieve optimum approximation. When possible, use a binocular loupe for accurate tissue alignment (Figure 8.2). Most facial lacerations can be closed in one layer.

Suturing Techniques

3/0–4/0 Vicryl or a similar absorbable suture is used for the nose, orbit, ears, and oral cavity.

4/0 Nylon is used for the skin.

To avoid damaging the skin edges with toothed forceps, a skin hook should be used to produce accurate wound apposition. A smooth wrist rotation will pass the curve of the needle through

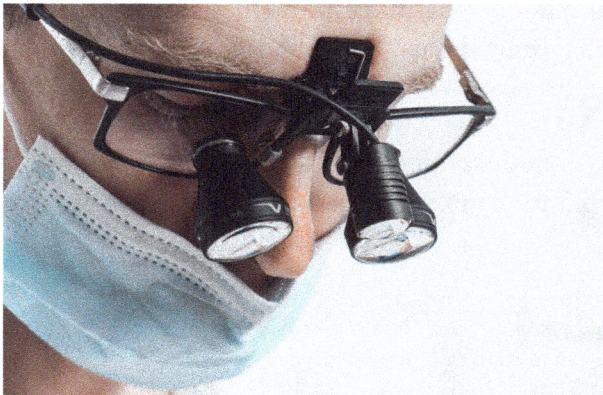

Figure 8.2 Binocular loupe for fine suturing.

the tissues and the suture material is then gently pulled through. Sutures can be placed in an interrupted or continuous fashion. Interrupted sutures give a superior aesthetic result, but careful continuous intradermal sutures can also give an aesthetic outcome. Sutures placed on the face should be approximately 1–2 mm from the skin margin and approximately 3 mm apart. The wound is closed in layers while avoiding overly tight knots. Lacerations in which the skin margins can be aligned without tension can be closed with a continuous technique. Irregular lacerations should be closed with an interrupted suture for the following reasons:

- If an area looks infected, it can be treated without having to open the entire wound by removing a few sutures in the hyperaemic area. After opening the margin, the wound is irrigated with warm water or saline and dressed with an antiseptic, such as povidone iodine gauze or a Manuka dressing. This will allow the wound to drain, the infection will resolve, and keep the scar small. Systemic antibiotics only need to be given to eliminate a spreading cellulitis. Topical antiseptic solutions can also be used as an adjunct to systemic antibiotics in wounds with signs of cellulitis.
- If the wound is closed by a continuous suture, partial removal of the suture is not possible and if infected, the entire suture will need to be removed as the wound will reopen. This results in a much larger scar.

Sutures should be removed after 5–7 days to minimise scarring. See Figure 8.3 for an example of a wound that required fine suturing in layers.

Repair Guidance

After the wound edges are sutured, a small amount of antiseptic is applied: povidone iodine, which inhibits prostaglandin-induced

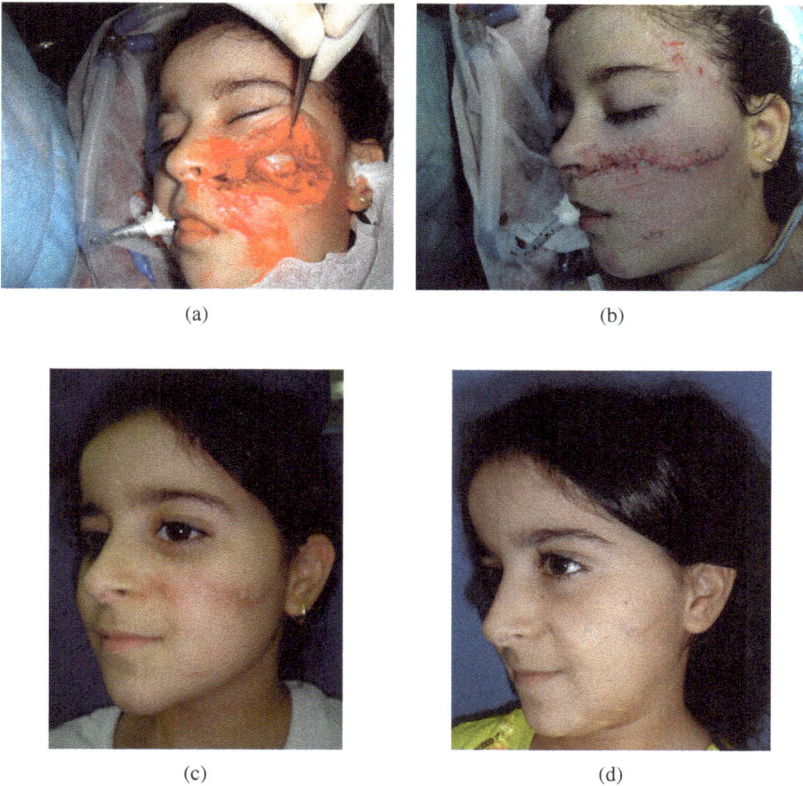

Figure 8.3　(a) and (b) A blast laceration, carefully debrided and finely sutured in layers (Misrata, Libya 2011); (c) Eight-week follow-up; (d) One year later.

inflammation to numb the painful area, or chlorhexidine digluconate, which is an antiseptic. It is then covered with dry gauze.

- The dressing can be removed two days later.
- The patient can shower and wash the face as usual the day after the repair.
- Facial injuries cause the tissues to swell and so the patient should be warned that the face will be swollen for several days.
- The patient should also avoid bending and heavy lifting for several days, which also promote facial swelling.

Combat Wound Dressings

- Combat wounds with a high level of contamination need early cleansing, then dressing or surgical closure to avoid infection.
- The problems with combat wounds are potentially their large size and the heavy drainage of blood and serum. Such wounds should be assessed for necrosis and infection, which will require moisture-retentive dressings that include hydrogels, hydrocolloids, foams, and alginates.
- Antimicrobial impregnated dressings are useful in superficially infected wounds.

Moist Wound Healing

Wounds covered with moisture-retentive dressings or ointments heal faster than exposed or gauze-covered wounds.

The moisture in a wound contains proteins and cytokines that facilitate autolytic debridement, angiogenesis that is the formation of granulation tissue, and keratinocyte migration which is responsible for the formation of the overlying skin.[2]

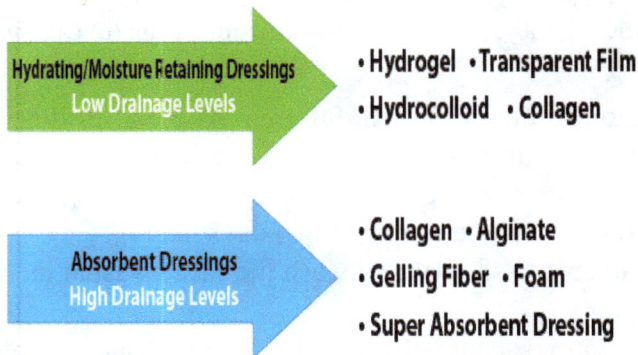

Figure 8.4 Types of dressing.

Credit: Eula Reynolds RN, MSN, CWS, DAPWCA, Director of Clinical Education, DermaRite Industries.

If a deep wound is left open to the air, a hard scab of dried blood and exudate forms. The scab forms from dried blood as the body's self-defence to protect the injured area. However, this is different from eschar, which is necrotic tissue that must be removed by debridement as it predisposes the wound to further infection.

Choice of Dressing

There are innumerable dressings to choose from (see Figure 8.4). Most important in a war setting is to have access to dressings that are cheap and readily available, for example simple gauze.

Analgesia

The patient's pain must be controlled by analgesics.

Oral analgesia:
- Ibuprofen 400 mg, 8 hourly or prn.
- Diclofenac sodium 50 mg, orally two or three times in 24 h.

Narcotic analgesics:
- Fentanyl 0.05–0.1 mg, IM or IV.
- Tramadol for moderate to severe pain, 50–100 mg orally every 4–6 h.
- Morphine 10–20 mg × 3, oral or IM daily.

Review of Key Points

- A moist wound healing environment under the dressing is now recommended as dry dressings result in wound tissue damage.
- Dressings should be left in place for up to two days or more in order to avoid interrupting the healing process.

- All trauma wounds should undergo debridement and a thorough irrigation before primary closure. The aim of debridement is to remove all contaminated and devitalised tissue.
- A primary suture is not indicated in heavily contaminated wounds, where the risk of infection is high. The wound should be debrided and dressed, and suturing is carried out later when the wound is free of inflammation and discharge.
- Wounds should not be allowed to heal by secondary intention. This healing is slow and leads to contractures, scarring, and restriction of movement and may require reconstruction with a skin graft.

References

1. Brown A. When is wound cleansing necessary and what solution should be used? *Nursing Times* [online]. 2018;114(9):42–45.
2. Broussard KC, Powers JG. Wound dressings: Selecting the most appropriate type. *Am J Clin Dermatol.* 2013 Dec;14(6):449–459. doi: 10.1007/s40257-013-0046-4. PMID: 24062083.

Chapter 9

Post-Traumatic Stress Disorder

Muhammad M. Rahman

Introduction

The World Health Organisation created the International Statistical Classification of Diseases and Related Health Problems (ICD) to classify mental health illnesses. Here, trauma is described as a single event or a series of events that threaten or harm the individual physically or emotionally. An acute stress disorder (ASD) describes the effects of trauma that occur immediately after the event, whereas a post-traumatic stress disorder (PTSD) refers to long-term effects.

ASD is a transient disorder developing in an individual with no apparent mental health problems and is caused by exceptional physical or mental stress factors. The reaction to the stress factors usually subsides within a few hours or days depending on the individual's vulnerability and coping capacity. The symptoms of ASD are mixed but usually start with the individual becoming dazed and disorientated. This can be followed by dissociation from their surroundings or by agitation. Signs of anxiety, such as sweating, flushing, and tachycardia, are also commonly present. In some cases, amnesia of the episode can occur.

PTSD can be described as the long-term effects of an exceptionally catastrophic or threatening episode which would be likely to cause distress to almost anyone. There may be predisposing factors such as a previous history of neurotic illness. Another difference between ASD and PTSD is that ASD is characteristic for repeated flashbacks of the traumatic event that perpetuate a host of effects, such as emotional blunting, with detachment and avoidance of situations that are reminiscent of the trauma event. There are also heightened startle reactions as well as insomnia.

Anxiety and depression are common in PTSD sufferers, which may lead to suicidal intent. In a war environment, PTSD is thought to mainly affect soldiers; however, civilians may also be affected. While doctors and surgeons may have a greater stress threshold given their training, they are not immune to mental health disorders.

Diagnosing and Treating PTSD

Psychological Management of PTSD

Albert Ellis was an American psychologist (Figure 9.1) who, in 1955, developed rational emotive behavioural therapy (REBT). He is generally considered to be one of the originators of a shift in psychotherapy and the second-most influential psychotherapist in history. Carl Rogers was ranked first and Sigmund Freud was ranked third.[1,2]

'No individual — not even Freud himself — has had a greater impact on modern psychotherapy'. 'We aim to understand how PTSD develops from exposure to a war environment'.

The diagnosis of psychological illnesses is very subjective as there are few biological markers that define the disorder.

The National Institute for Health and Care Excellence (NICE) classification of PTSD lists the types of traumatic events that are likely to cause the disorder, which include serious accidents, physical

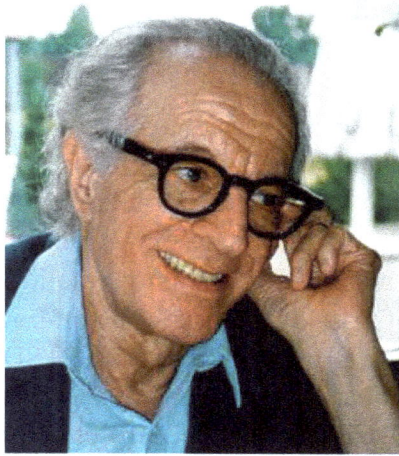

Figure 9.1 Albert Ellis 1913–2007. Credit: Dr. Albert Ellis and The Albert Ellis Institute, NY.

assault, work-related exposure to trauma, and torture. All these factors fit the war environment but can apply equally to civilians and health-care workers. There are several symptoms associated with functional disorders, including flashbacks, depression, and social events, such as a state of increased psychological and physiological tension (hyperarousal), social avoidance, and problems maintaining relationships.

For the prevention of PTSD, individuals who have ASD are recommended to undergo treatment for trauma disorders, cognitive processing therapy, and narrative exposure therapy. Treatment for adults is mainly cognitive behavioural therapy (CBT) for those who have presented with PTSD a month after the initial traumatic event. It is important that the CBT given is delivered by a trained practitioner. It is also recommended that the patient receives at least eight sessions and part of the therapy should include strategies for managing a strong response to flashbacks and traumatic memories. A deeper processing of emotions is also required in order that the patient can self-manage feelings such as shame, guilt, loss, and anger. These are the first steps of the individual's recovery. Further to this, sufferers should then focus on adaptive functioning for work environments and social relationships. With severe traumatic events, there is always the chance that memories can be triggered, so even if the patient can manage their trauma, booster sessions should be considered before the anniversary of the event.

A recent psychotherapy is eye movement desensitisation and reprocessing, as a means of dampening emotionally charged traumatic memories of past events. It is a non-traditional school of psychotherapy, especially used for treating PTSD after experiences such as military combat, physical assault and rape, or car accidents.

To accompany CBT, selective serotonin reuptake inhibitors (SSRIs), such as Venlafaxine or Sertraline, can be administered. Antipsychotics such as Risperidone can be given if the SSRI drugs are ineffective and the patient suffers from disabling behaviour, such as hyperarousal.

Since 2018, NICE has recognised the need to screen children for PTSD symptoms. This comes with the reality of war in regions, such as the Middle East, where countries have had unrest lasting many years. Civilians living in such war environments, refugees, and asylum seekers should also be considered. It is recommended that refugees and asylum seekers are screened within a month of leaving a war zone.

For children and young people of ages from 6 to 17, CBT group therapy is helpful in that children will meet others with similar experiences away from the trauma and other stress factors, so that they may be able to benefit together. However, the treatment needs to be adapted for their age and parents and guardians must also be involved.

PTSD in Military Personnel

The 2013 edition of the DSM-5 highlights the stigma for military personnel as they believe the word 'disorder' makes soldiers who suffer with PTSD symptoms less likely to seek help.[1]

The military wanted to change the name from post-traumatic stress *'disorder'* to post traumatic stress *'injury'*; however, this was rejected with the reasoning that the military should instead change their management so that help is more available and that soldiers do not feel embarrassed to seek it.

Soldiers are trained to be effective in a war environment by desensitisation and by mental and physical hardening. All forms of scenarios are presented to them, including suicide bombs, to prepare them for the most traumatic events. One study has demonstrated that PTSD preventative interventions given to US soldiers three months before deployment to Iraq in 2011 did not have any significant difference compared to the control group which suffered PTSD 12 months post deployment.[3] This implies that despite preparations made to prevent PTSD, the events that occur in a war environment are traumatic enough to result in developing the disorder.

Military personnel often come from peaceful countries with stable environments and are mobilised to countries such as Afghanistan and Iraq which have become destroyed, lawless, and dangerous from long-lasting warfare. There, they regularly witness events not just of direct violence but the impact of war on civilians and the distress caused. As these military personnel return to their homes, there can be problems with reintegration socially and mentally. A study of 1,710 British veterans of the Afghanistan and Iraq wars demonstrated that their experience of military action was a risk factor for their return to the UK and there was no difference between the effects of their combat and non-combat roles.[4] Violent behaviour observed by these veterans while on duty strongly affected their mental health risk factors, which included PTSD and alcohol abuse, suggesting that those who went to a war zone had been influenced to become violent even when they were non-combatant.

PTSD is associated with various mental health issues, including ASD and depression, which is a dangerous mix that culminates in a complex mental state. While the recommended treatment is 8 to 12 sessions of CBT, studies have shown that those British veterans given six weeks of treatment post military action showed reduced PTSD severity, reduced anxiety, depression, and anger when followed up after a year.[5] Veterans that responded poorly to PTSD treatment within the first six weeks were found to have functional impairment and alcohol problems when followed up after a year. This demonstrated that treatment for PTSD should be considered beyond a year and although beneficial, many cases can be complicated by alcohol and such patients will need more help.

PTSD in Terrorised Civilians from a Peaceful Environment

PTSD has always been associated with the military; however, the largest population exposed to traumatic events can be civilians. Unlike military personnel, civilians are not trained or prepared physically and mentally for traumatic events, such as terrorist attacks in non-war environments. The 9/11 attacks were a series of four coordinated terrorist attacks by the Islamic terrorist group al-Qaeda against the United States on the morning of September 11, 2001 (see Figures 9.2 and 9.3). The attacks resulted in nearly 3,000 fatalities, over 25,000 injuries, and substantial long-term health consequences. In addition, there was at least USD 10 billion in property damage. The 9/11 attack is the single deadliest terrorist attack in human history and the single deadliest incident for firefighters and law enforcement officers in the history of the United States, with 343 and 72 killed, respectively. This also led to PTSD and functional impairment that was present four years after the initial event.[6] Although patients show a gradual decline in PTSD, there was a considerable increase in suicidal ideation and days taken off work. The biggest risk factor was found to be the loss of a relative or close friend. The attack was very sudden which is also a factor, and the witnesses to the event were unprepared, making the experience more traumatic. Other terrorist attacks have

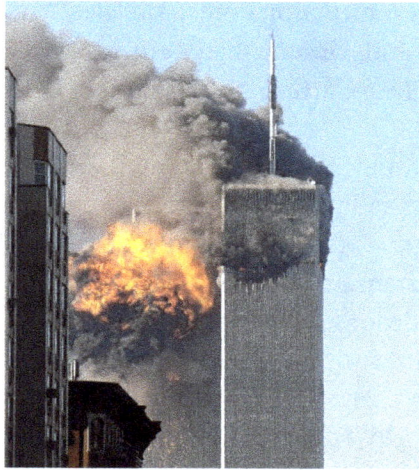

Figure 9.2 United Airlines Flight 175 crashes into the south tower of the World Trade Centre during the September 11 attacks.

Source: https://commons.wikimedia.org/wiki/File:UA_Flight_175_hits_WTC_south_tower_9-11.jpeg. Attribution: Robert J. Fisch.

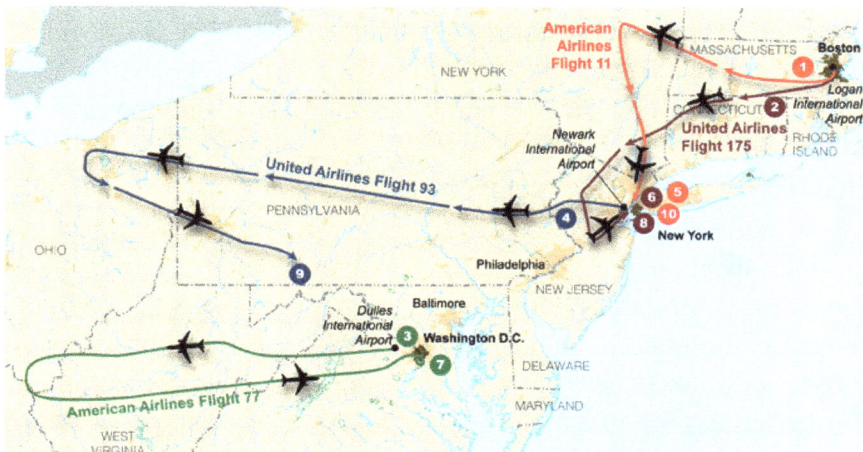

Figure 9.3 Flight paths of the four planes used on September 11.

occurred since 9/11 in major cities, such as Madrid and London, equally shocking and violent in nature to the civilians; however, sufferers were able to return to a relatively normal setting and ordered lifestyle.

The greatest casualties of war are civilians, particularly in long-term conflicts such as in Syria and Iraq. Compared to terror attacks in peaceful settings, wars in the Middle East have been long lasting and devastating because of mass shelling and bombing. This can be by tanks, planes, drones, etc. Furthermore, the various armies and factions involved means that there is a lot of violence and a constant military or rebel presence. While the 9/11 attack was large enough to collapse the World Trade Centre, the surrounding infrastructure of Manhattan was undamaged, which is different to the situation in the Middle East where towns and cities are flattened. The damage to society is large scale in that many lose their jobs, children may not be able to go to school, and there is a constant threat of violence. This emphasises that there are traumatic events that will be experienced by civilians in a non-war environment where the likelihood of structured treatment is low. For instance, the situation for civilians in some parts of the Middle East is so severe that they will do everything in their power to escape despite the risks. A study of Middle Eastern asylum seekers that were screened and psychoanalysed for PTSD revealed that 96% experienced more than one major traumatic event and that 33% had PTSD.[7] Furthermore, 39% had psychiatric morbidity. The study revealed that PTSD was strongly associated with the level of war trauma experienced and the length of time spent in refugee camps. A larger-scale study of Middle Eastern and African asylum seekers to Italy details the traumas suffered by the cohort. Of the asylum seekers, 44% suffered from PTSD with 68% being either physically or mentally tortured.[8] Furthermore, 66% of asylum seekers had witnessed someone being physically harmed, 61% witnessed torture or murder, 38% shelling, and 37% witnessed sexual abuse. While many of these categories are not direct abuse, witnessing such events is highly traumatic.

Regarding direct trauma, 60% were beaten, 57% imprisoned, 43% kidnapped or taken hostage, 37% knifed, 37% injured indirectly from landmines or combat, and 35% sexually abused or raped. People suffering the strongest effects of PTSD and related disorders are likely to be those that were physically abused. The survey also revealed that 58% were forced into hiding, 56% were ill and had no access to medical care, 49% were missing a family member or friend, 49% had a family member injured, 47% were forced to separate from family, 46% confined to their homes, and 38% had their property damaged or looted. These are examples of social and emotional loss likely to be associated with depression despite not being victims of physical harm.

Conclusion

The differences between military and civilian experiences of trauma are very distinct. Military personnel are trained and desensitised before military action. They are trained to be in dangerous situations and expect to experience trauma. Soldiers are also armed, so they have a sense of control in dangerous situations and the ability to protect themselves. Civilians have no control during terror events; they are only able to shelter where possible. Furthermore, the military are deployed for a limited time, whereas civilians may not have the option to flee the war zone, exposing them to sustained trauma.

It is also important to consider non-military workers, such as surgeons, nurses, and aid workers, and how they cope in war environments. While medical staff would have witnessed injuries, they may not have seen such large numbers of casualties, as when a bomb explodes in a crowded area. It is evident that despite conditioning and training, there is still a strong possibility that experiencing war trauma will be a major cause of PTSD and associated mental disorders.

References

1. American Psychiatric Association. Diagnostic and Statistical Manual of Mental Disorders. 5th ed. Arlington, VA: American Psychiatric Publishing, 2013.
2. Pyne JM, Constans JI, Nanney JT, Wiederhold MD, Gibson DP, Kimbrell T, Kramer TL, Pitcock JA, Han X, Williams DK, Chartrand D, Gevirtz RN, Spira J, Wiederhold BK, McCraty R, McCune TR. Heart rate variability and cognitive bias feedback interventions to prevent post-deployment PTSD: Results from a randomized controlled trial. *Mil Med.* 2019 Jan 1;184(1–2):e124–e132. doi: 10.1093/milmed/usy171. PMID: 30020511; PMCID: PMC6751385.
3. MacManus D, Dickson H, Short R, Burdett H, Kwan J, Jones M, Hull L, Wessely S, Fear NT. Risk and protective factors for offending among UK Armed Forces personnel after they leave service: A data linkage study. *Psychol Med.* 2021 Jan;51(2):236–243. doi: 10.1017/S0033291719003131. Epub 2019 Nov 29. PMID: 31779726.
4. Rona RJ, Burdett H, Bull S, Jones M, Jones N, Greenberg N, Wessely S, Fear NT. Prevalence of PTSD and other mental disorders in UK service personnel by time since end of deployment: A meta-analysis. *BMC Psychiatry.* 2016 Sep 22;16(1):333. doi: 10.1186/s12888-016-1038-8. PMID: 27659728; PMCID: PMC5034433.
5. Murphy D, Spencer-Harper L, Carson C, Palmer E, Hill K, Sorfleet N, Wessely S, Busuttil W. Long-term responses to treatment in UK veterans with military-related PTSD: An observational study. *BMJ Open.* 2016 Sep 16;6(9):e011667. doi: 10.1136/bmjopen-2016-011667. PMID: 27638494; PMCID: PMC5030535.
6. Neria Y, Wickramaratne P, Olfson M, Gameroff MJ, Pilowsky DJ, Lantigua R, Shea S, Weissman MM. Mental and physical health consequences of the September 11, 2001 (9/11) attacks in primary care: A longitudinal study. *J Trauma Stress.* 2013 Feb;26(1):45–55. doi: 10.1002/jts.21767. Epub 2013 Jan 14. PMID: 23319335; PMCID: PMC3685149.
7. Fino E, Mema D, Russo PM. War trauma exposed refugees and posttraumatic stress disorder: The moderating role of trait resilience. *J Psychosom Res.* 2020 Feb;129:109905. doi: 10.1016/j.jpsychores.2019.109905. Epub 2019 Dec 16. PMID: 31869693.
8. Rodolico A, Vaccino N, Riso MC, Concerto C, Aguglia E, Signorelli MS. Prevalence of post-traumatic stress disorder among asylum seekers in Italy: A population-based survey in Sicily. *J Immigr Minor Health.* 2020 Jun;22(3):634–638. doi: 10.1007/s10903-019-00948-9. PMID: 31863404.

Chapter 10

Terrorism and Craniofacial Injuries

Eran Regev and Rephael Zeltser

Introduction

Terrorism is unlawful aggression, usually urban, which can become widespread indiscriminate violence creating panic in civilian populations. The aims can be social, political, racist, or religious. There is little difference between the casualties of terrorism in a 'wealth and peace' environment and those of violence in an 'austere and war' zone (see Introduction to this book for explanation of this terminology). Currently, significant numbers suffer identical ballistic and penetrating wounds in both environments. From a medical emergency standpoint, in austere and war zones, there is the expectancy that a large number of casualties can arrive at one time and the likelihood that they will suffer from similar injuries. Terrorist acts in wealth and peace environments are sudden with emergency services often unprepared to deal with large numbers of casualties with uncommon injuries; an example is the Bataclan theatre terrorist attack in Paris in 2015, which resulted in the deaths of 130 people along with 413 injured individuals from gunshot wounds. A similar attack occurred in Las Vegas in 2017, where 60 died and 411 were injured from assault rifle fire that would be more in line with injuries in a war zone.

Other terrorist attacks that occurred in wealth and peace settings include the Madrid bombings in 2004 with 191 fatalities and over 2,000 injuries and the Manchester arena bombing in 2017 with 22 deaths and 138 injured. Explosive devices used in terrorist attacks often include nails or other shrapnel, and the injuries can be significant, especially in the face and hands. Dobson *et al.* found that only 16% of all war injuries involved the maxillofacial area.[1]

Terrorism casualties require to be managed by clinical emergency care, hence the need for specialist medical personnel and paramedical services to compliment untrained healthcare providers. This chapter highlights the importance of the presence of a craniofacial consultant surgeon right from the beginning of treating trauma cases. However, for the purpose of this book, it also serves to illustrate the importance of educating non-specialists about crucial craniofacial problems for when this is not possible. Furthermore, the 2002 Beirut ammonium nitrate storage explosion, a non-terrorism incident, resulted in the death of 218 people and over 7,500 injuries from the blast and shrapnel, similar to what would be expected in a war zone, thus highlighting the importance of training.

Injuries in Israel

The five principal types of terrorism injury are:

(1) stone-related injuries;
(2) stab wounds;
(3) gunshot wounds;
(4) blast injuries;
(5) burns.

Stones

Stones have been used in civilian uprisings and riots for centuries and are still a popular weapon, causing severe injuries during the First Palestinian Intifada (1987–1993). Of the injuries suffered by Israeli troops in 1987–1989, 62% were caused by stones.[2,3] Between 2000 and 2004, the characteristics of political violence in Israel changed to explosions and gunfire, and in that period, only 13% of the injuries were caused by stones. However, a distinction can be made between two types of victims: those who stood facing the rioters at a 'stone-throwing distance' and those who were in a car moving towards the stone thrower.

The first type of victims was composed almost exclusively of army troops who were facing rioters. Heering described 370 skull, face, and neck injuries among 611 soldiers wounded by stones, 70 of whom sustained jaw injuries.[4] The vast majority of the head and neck injuries in their study were graded as light injuries; however, the authors comment on the lack of protective equipment that the soldiers should have been wearing.

The second type of victims includes drivers and passengers of motor vehicles. When a stone hits a car moving at 40–50 mi/h, the velocity at impact is the sum of the car velocity and the stone's velocity. Therefore, the severity of injuries sustained even by having a small stone thrown at a moving car can be substantial. The facial fractures are usually open and comminuted. In addition, a stone often shatters the car window before hitting the occupant, adding lacerations by the glass fragments. The head and neck are the areas most frequently affected by stoning because they are at window level and unprotected by the door. Drivers of left-hand-drive cars are almost always injured on the left side of the face and passengers on the right side. Stone throwing also increases the risk of secondary injury from a driver's loss of control, when swerving to avoid being hit results in collision with another vehicle or driving off the road.

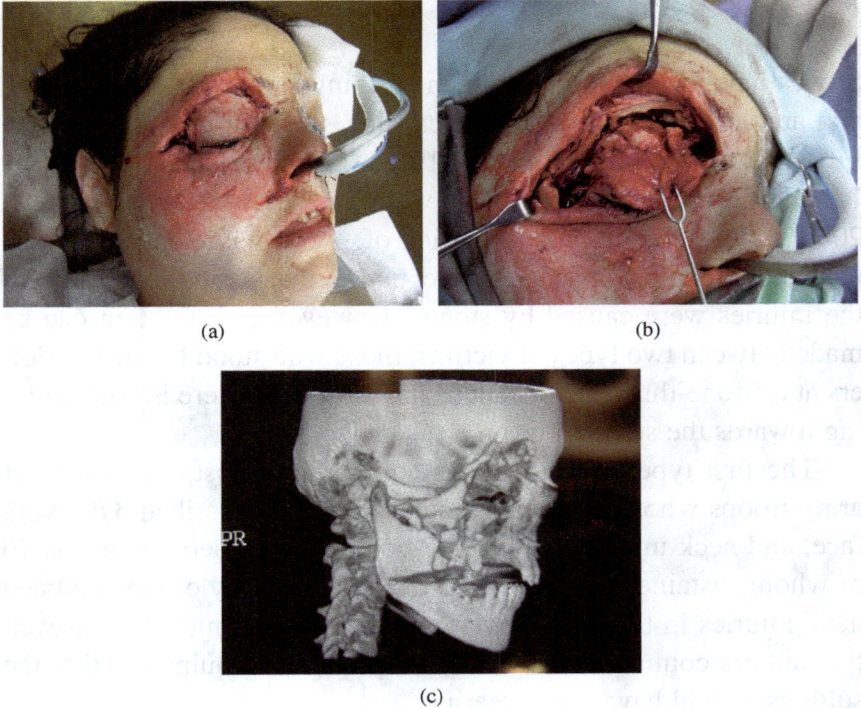

(a)

(b)

(c)

Figure 10.1 (a) Blunt stone injury of the right orbit showing a peri-orbital laceration; (b) Flap which is pulled down reveals the globe of the eye and the contents of the orbit. The fractured lateral and superior rims of the orbital bone are
visible and can be seen in the computed tomography (CT) scan; (c) CT scan
showing the comminution of the coronoid process of the ramus of the mandible
and the adjacent fractured maxilla and orbital floor.

Treatment

The result of a stone injury is blunt trauma on the facial soft tissues.

Fractures caused by stones are comminuted with soft-tissue lacerations (Figure 10.1), and treatment should include debridement
with preservation of tissue and bone reconstruction by intermaxillary fixation (IMF) or open reduction with internal fixation (ORIF).
A car occupant injured by a stone may suffer comminuted fractures
of the orbit, zygoma, and coronoid process.

Stab Wounds

Hanoch *et al.* reviewed 154 patients who were stabbed in acts of political violence in Israel between 1987 and 1994.[5] Unlike in 'civilian' stabbings, about half of these victims sustained multiple wounds. The most common site was the posterior right thorax, though the head and neck were involved in 49 patients. Stabbings accounted for fewer than 3% of the maxillofacial injuries. In some societies, civilian stab wounds are much more common; for instance, in South Africa, 393 cases of head and neck stab wounds were reported in a period of 21 months.[6] A study reported that stab wounds accounted for 26% of the trauma patients admitted to an emergency department in another hospital.[7] The major vessels of the head and neck, the trachea and the oesophagus have been the target areas for stabbing attacks. Stab wounds in the face are rare and, unlike the neck injuries, are not life threatening.

Treatment

Deep neck stab injuries are investigated for damage to the platysma. If the patient is haemodynamically stable, with no active bleeding, or if the knife is impacted in the wound, angiography or CT angiography should be performed. This displays the path of the blade and possible damage to blood vessels prior to removal of the weapon. The advantage of angiography is the ability to embolise bleeding vessels and avoid a blind surgical neck exploration.

Gunshot Injuries

(See also Chapters 12 and 13).

Firearm injuries are not unique to military activity, and the vast majority of the literature is about civilian incidents.[8,9] The velocity of the bullet is the main factor for distinguishing the pattern of injury. Other important factors are the bullet type and shape, proximity of the victim to the muzzle, protective equipment that the bullet has penetrated, and tissues encountered. Powers and Robertson have discussed common myths relating to ballistics in the area of oral and maxillofacial surgery.[10] They concluded that tissue injury is caused by the design of the bullet and its energy upon striking the tissue and that the velocity alone cannot be the basis for the lesion. For example, a bullet from a low-velocity handgun shot from a short distance and hitting the facial or jaw bones may cause more damage than a bullet from a high-velocity

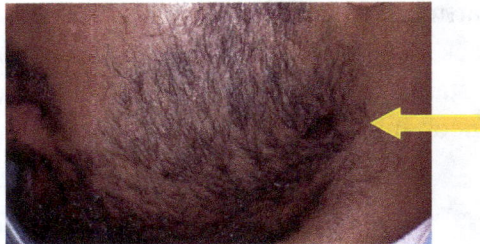

(a)

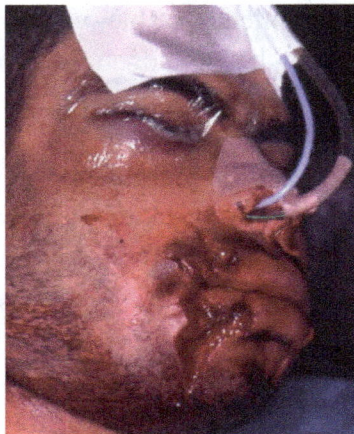

(b)

Figure 10.2   (a) Gunshot entry wound in the lower-left face; (b) Gunshot exit wound.

rifle fired from a long distance and penetrating only soft tissue. The Israel National Trauma Registry recorded that, of the gunshot wounds from 2000 to 2004, 25% of them involved the head and neck (Figure 10.2).[11]

Treatment

As the goal is to preserve life, the advanced trauma life support (ATLS) protocol is applied first (see Chapter 2). Gunshot wounds to the maxillofacial region may severely damage the upper airway and require emergency endotracheal intubation. Sometimes, this is not feasible because of massive bleeding or anatomical distortion, and therefore a cricothyroidotomy is performed. Once the airway is established, haemorrhage should be controlled. If a major neck vessel is bleeding profusely, local pressure should be applied until the patient is taken to the operating room for exploration.

A common surgical dictum is 'treat the wound, not the weapon' i.e. treatment is based on the presentation of the wound and not on the type of weapon or projectile. The two treatment protocols for gunshot injuries are immediate or delayed reconstruction.[12,13] Immediate reconstruction is defined as initial treatment of a wound, with the intention to definitively manage all aspects of the injury. The aim is to close the wound in such a way that both hard and soft tissues are restored. This may require the introduction of rigid fixation and then immediate bone grafts and tissue flaps to close soft and hard tissue defects.

In the delayed reconstruction protocol, the initial treatment includes stabilisation of bone injuries, maximum tissue preservation, and closure of the wounds with local mucosa and skin. Necrotic tissue and bone fragments that are not attached to the periosteum or soft tissues are excised. Since the maxillofacial region has an excellent blood supply, any bone, teeth, or soft tissue that has a chance to remain vital is not removed. Final reconstruction is attempted after oedema has resolved and soft tissue covers the wound. This may be carried out several weeks or months later in one or several stages (Figure 10.3).

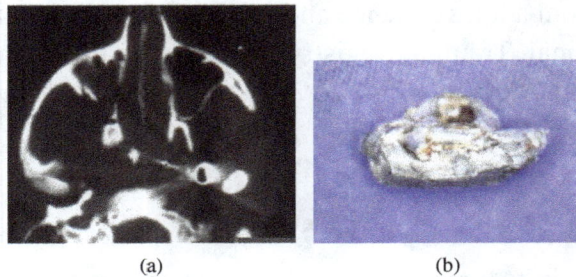

(a)   (b)

Figure 10.3   (a) Bullet in the left infra temporal fossa; (b) Retrieved bullet.

Explosions and Blast Injuries

Among the many and varied weapons that terrorists have used, the most common ones in recent years are those involving explosives. Effects of the detonation can be devastating. An aerial bomb may contain as much as one ton of explosive charges encased in metal.

A bomb explosion involves the sudden transformation of a solid or liquid material into gas, generating a blast wave that spreads out from a point source. The blast wave consists of two parts: the initial shock wave of high pressure, followed closely by a blast wind. The damage produced by the blast wave decreases with distance.[14] When the explosion occurs in a confined space, like a bus, the blast wave is reflected back from the walls, producing increased mortality and morbidity.[15,16]

The wounds caused by a bomb explosion are multiple and grossly contaminated. The common injuries are a combination of bruises, abrasions, lacerations, and superficial wounds. Facial fractures are multiple and serious.

There are four components of blast injury effects:

(1) **Primary:** The direct effect of pressure as the high explosive wave impacts on hollow body surfaces.
(2) **Secondary:** The effects of projectiles.
(3) **Tertiary:** The effect due to the blast wind propelling a victim against a stationary object.

(4) **Quaternary:** All other effects, including burns, asphyxia, and exposure to toxic inhalants.

The maxillofacial region is affected by the secondary, tertiary, and quaternary stages of the blast injury. The only part of the head and neck region affected by the primary injury is the eardrum which is a hollow organ sensitive to the overpressure wave when the victim is in proximity to the explosion.

An animal model developed by Wang *et al.* showed that the effect of the blast wave from a spherical explosion causes extensive wounds to soft tissue, skin, and muscle.[17] The bones of the facial skeleton suffer splinter fractures and the fracture sites become concave.

The consensus is that the secondary explosive mechanism causes the majority of the maxillofacial injuries (Figure 10.4). Shuker describes injury by blast wave and that acceleration, spalling, and implosion are factors that determine the amount of damage caused (Figure 10.5). Improvised suicide bombs detonated in Israel are not usually larger than 5–10 kg.[18] To enhance their effect of these explosives, many metal objects were added,

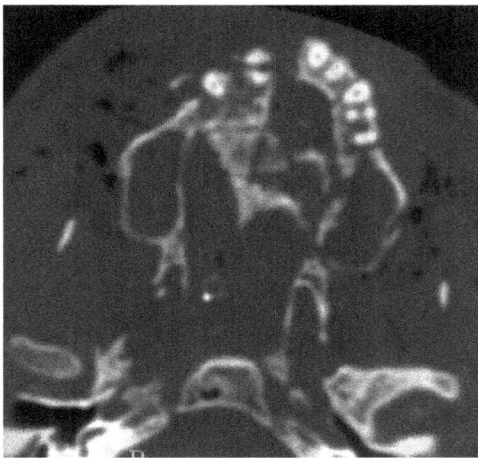

Figure 10.4   Blast destruction of the maxilla.

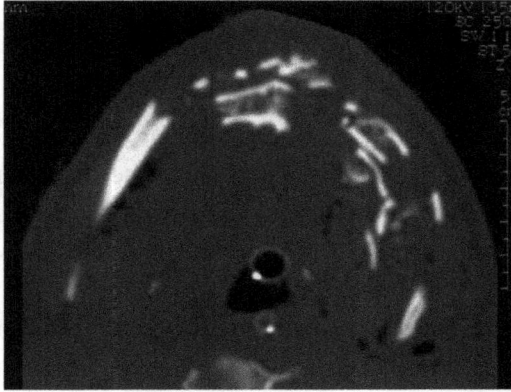

Figure 10.5   Blast destruction of the mandible.

including bolts, nails, screws, and ball bearings. Propelled by the explosive detonation, these projectiles hit numerous victims in the vicinity. At a velocity of 50 ft/s (17 m/s), skin is easily lacerated and at 400 ft/s (133 m/s), serious wounds are caused by deeper penetration into the body.[19] Depending on the distance from the centre of the explosion, the projectiles can penetrate the hard or soft tissues of the craniofacial region. Foreign objects can be projected into critical anatomical locations, such as a bolt in the brain after shattering the orbital walls, nails in the orbit, and a metal ball in cervical spine (Figures 10.6 and 10.7).

These injuries are similar to those caused by pellets from a high-energy shotgun. The projectiles behave like high-velocity missiles causing cavitation and damage to adjacent tissues.

Figure 10.8 illustrates how not all the projectiles come from inside the explosive device. This shows a wristwatch which was torn from the bomber's wrist by the blast wind.

Treatment

If lengthy procedures are contraindicated or the patient is oedematous, early maxillofacial intervention should be limited to stabilisation

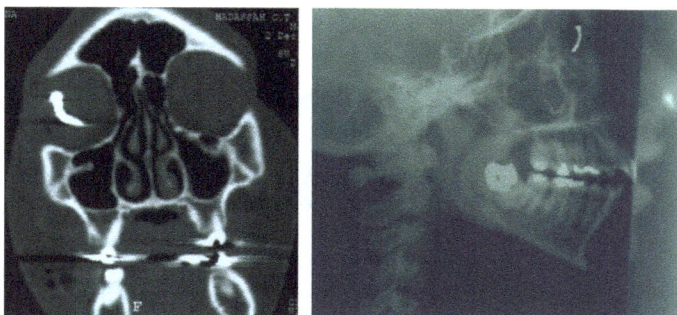

Figure 10.6   Nail embedded in the right eyeball from blast with complete loss of sight.

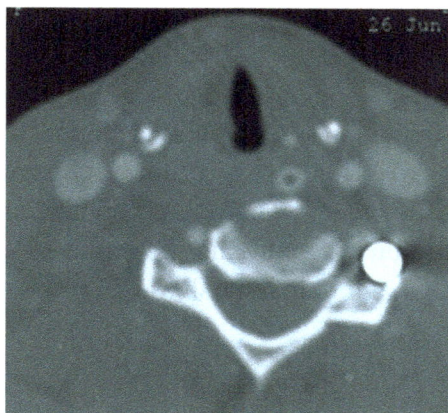

Figure 10.7   Metal sphere in the cervical spine.

of bone segments, such as intermaxillary fixation and interosseous plating and packing of soft-tissue wounds.

As a general rule for extensive blast injuries, the initial treatment includes bone stabilisation, usually with intermaxillary fixation, hard- and soft-tissue preservation, and an attempt to close all the wounds.

As the head and neck region has excellent vascularity, apparently unsalvageable tissue will often be viable. Soft-tissue wounds, lacerations, and abrasions may be contaminated with foreign materials as

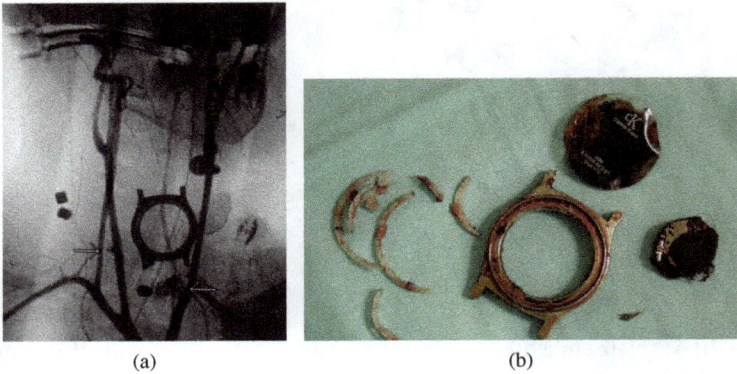

(a)   (b)

Figure 10.8   (a) CT angiogram showing the blast implosion of a watch in the bomber's chest; (b) Retrieved wristwatch and blast particles.

well as pieces of human tissue and blood. Thorough and repeated debridement and irrigation with copious amounts of water or saline should be performed prior to any primary closure which may be delayed when the wound margins are too oedematous to close. Embedded foreign objects should not be removed unless the risk of leaving them in is greater than the risk associated with their removal.

Burns

The blast overpressure wave is the sudden pressure wave after an explosion caused by the released energy. The heat wave travels at the speed of sound and causes injuries due to fire and gas inhalation to the face, eyes, oral tissues, and upper respiratory system. Burns of various degrees are encountered in combination with other injury patterns, as seen in Figure 10.9, showing a victim of an explosion blast of a suicide bomb inside a bus.

Treatment

Burns call for special attention. One of the difficulties encountered in patients with facial burns is securing the endotracheal tube to the burnt

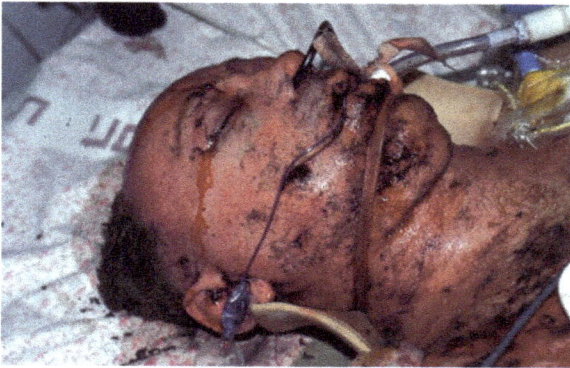

Figure 10.9   Overpressure blast explosive burn.

and oedematous skin. One solution is to secure the tube to the upper teeth, preferably the premolars, with flexible stainless-steel wire.[20]

Dealing with Large-Scale Incidents

Pre-Hospital Issues

In instances of terrorist acts, whereby the aim is to cause large number of casualties, the targets are buses and other crowded places, often in the centre of a city. Evacuation to a major hospital must be expedited. If an attack results in only a few casualties, the emergency medical services (EMS) can perform a 'scoop-and-run' evacuation to the nearest hospital. If there are many casualties, the scene can be chaotic and its management challenging. The area will rapidly fill with emergency medical teams, security, police personnel, and bystanders who may wish to help. The medical team leader at the site assumes control as the triage commander and assesses the condition of each victim and decides the treatment and evacuation priorities. The most seriously injured are sent to a level-1 trauma centre, while the other patients are evenly distributed among nearby hospitals. These decisions are made quickly as treatment is best rendered in a hospital and not in a pre-hospital setting.

Life-threatening conditions, such as a blocked airway or heavy bleeding, are immediately treated at the site or in transit to the hospital. There is no need for medical specialists at the site of the attack, though advance reports from the site or ambulances in transit should communicate with the receiving hospitals. In this way, the senior surgeon at the hospital is aware of the estimated number of victims, the severity of injuries, and whether an operating theatre is required immediately. Furthermore, maxillofacial trauma patients should be transported to a hospital with a maxillofacial surgery service.

Emergency Department

To minimise the confusion at a receiving hospital, rehearsed procedures should be in place for evacuation and distribution. Protocols for triage evaluation and treatment have been developed at the Hadassah University Hospital, Jerusalem in collaboration with the oral and maxillofacial surgery services.[21]

Treatment Protocol

The senior oral and maxillofacial surgeon should be present in the emergency department to assist the juniors in diagnosis, radiology priorities, and in operating room procedures. This surgeon should be involved in the initial evaluation and resuscitation of the victims who may have airway problems due to fractured jaws, aspirated fragments of bones and teeth, and massive oral and nasal bleeding.

The surgeon may also be needed to assist the anaesthetist with difficult intubation that requires securing the endotracheal tube to the teeth, as in the case of facial burns. Most endotracheal intubations are oral and performed by the EMS in the emergency department. For a thorough maxillofacial examination and for later surgical procedures, nasal intubation or a tracheostomy may be preferable, although not advised in an acute setting. The oral tube can be changed later, although nasal placement of an endotracheal tube is contraindicated in a patient with a closed head injury until a base of skull fracture is ruled out.

After the initial evaluation, imaging is essential for treatment planning. Plain X-rays can be obtained in the trauma room of the emergency department. However, if the head or neck of a patient is seriously injured, the required positioning for optimal radiographs may not be possible and would affect their quality. The ideal means for imaging facial injuries is a spiral CT scan with thin cuts and three-dimensional reconstructions, which provides the surgeons with a complete facial image within a few minutes and can be done with CT scans of the cervical spine, lungs, abdomen, and pelvis. This is only possible after securing the airway and ensuring hemodynamic stability.

Photographic documentation of any lesions is invaluable and helps confirm the identification of a patient who has been reported missing or taken to the operating theatre before being seen by the family. Photographs with cell phones are equally valuable for pre- and post-operative records, a task that can be assigned to a junior resident or student. Failure to keep full documentation of all injuries can lead to misdiagnosis.

An essential part of the acute protocol is to conduct debriefings at the end of the initial stage by the attending physician along with the residents.

Later, a secondary survey is conducted of all the maxillofacial patients with reviews of their imaging reports. A full-staff ward round is also performed the following day.

Conclusion

Ideally, an oral and maxillofacial surgeon should be present in the trauma team in the event of a multi-casualty incident.

The immediate concern with maxillofacial injuries is to secure the airway and arrest orofacial bleeding. After a thorough clinical examination, a cranial CT scan is essential for the detailed diagnosis of maxillofacial injuries.

Of the five types of injury recognised here, the characteristics of gunshot and stab wounds are similar to each other. Stones however, especially those thrown at a moving vehicle, can cause severe facial injuries. Of the four categories of blast injury, the secondary and tertiary categories affect the maxillofacial structures, although the primary blast may also cause eardrum and para-nasal sinus fractures and splinter fractures of the mandible.

Due to the complexity of multi-trauma damage, some maxillofacial injuries may be overlooked in the primary examination. As such, a structured protocol must include maxillofacial expertise after the initial normalisation and a post-operative tertiary survey the following day.

References

1. Dobson JE, Newell MJ, Shepherd JP. Trends in maxillofacial injuries in wartime (1914–1986). *Br J Oral Maxillofac Surg*. 1989 Dec;27(6):441–450. doi: 10.1016/s0266-4356(89)80001-4. PMID: 2688739.
2. Adler J, Golan E, Golan J, Yitzhaki M, Ben-Hur N. Terrorist bombing experience during 1975–1979. Casualties admitted to the Shaare Zedek Medical Center. *Isr J Med Sci*. 1983 Feb;19(2):189–193. PMID: 6841047.
3. Mintz Y, Shapira SC, Pikarsky AJ, Goitein D, Gertcenchtein I, Mor-Yosef S, Rivkind AI. The experience of one institution dealing with terror: The El Aqsa Intifada riots. *Isr Med Assoc J*. 2002 Jul;4(7):554–556. PMID: 12120471.
4. Heering SL, Shohat T, Lerman Y, Danon YL. The epidemiology of injuries sustained by Israeli troops during the unrest in the territories administered by Israel, 1987–1989. *Isr J Med Sci*. 1992 Jun;28(6):341–344. PMID: 1607268.
5. Hanoch J, Feigin E, Pikarsky A, Kugel C, Rivkind A. Stab wounds associated with terrorist activities in Israel. *JAMA*. 1996 Aug 7;276(5):388–390. PMID: 8683817.
6. Apffelstaedt JP, Müller R. Results of mandatory exploration for penetrating neck trauma. *World J Surg*. 1994 Nov–Dec;18(6):917–919; Discussion 920. doi: 10.1007/BF00299107. PMID: 7846919.
7. Hudson DA. Impacted knife injuries of the face. *Br J Plast Surg*. 1992 Apr;45(3):222–224. doi: 10.1016/0007-1226(92)90082-9. PMID: 1596663.
8. Chen AY, Stewart MG, Raup G. Penetrating injuries of the face. *Otolaryngol Head Neck Surg*. 1996 Nov;115(5):464–470. doi: 10.1177/01945998-9611500519. PMID: 8903449.
9. Hollier L, Grantcharova EP, Kattash M. Facial gunshot wounds: A 4-year experience. *J Oral Maxillofac Surg*. 2001 Mar;59(3):277–282. doi: 10.1053/joms.2001.20989. PMID: 11243609.

10. Powers DB, Robertson OB. Ten common myths of ballistic injuries. *Oral Maxillofac Surg Clin North Am.* 2005 Aug;17(3):251–259, v. doi: 10.1016/j. coms.2005.05.001. PMID: 18088782.

11. Peleg K, Aharonson-Daniel L, Stein M, Michaelson M, Kluger Y, Simon D, Noji EK; Israeli Trauma Group (ITG). Gunshot and explosion injuries: characteristics, outcomes, and implications for care of terror-related injuries in Israel. *Ann Surg.* 2004 Mar;239(3):311–318. doi: 10.1097/01. sla.0000114012.84732.be. PMID: 15075646; PMCID: PMC1356227.

12. Motamedi MH. Primary treatment of penetrating injuries to the face. *J Oral Maxillofac Surg.* 2007 Jun;65(6):1215–1218. doi: 10.1016/j. joms.2007.03.001. PMID: 17517308.

13. Ueeck BA. Penetrating injuries to the face: Delayed versus primary treatment--considerations for delayed treatment. *J Oral Maxillofac Surg.* 2007 Jun;65(6):1209–1214. doi: 10.1016/j.joms.2006.10.078. PMID: 17517307.

14. DePalma RG, Burris DG, Champion HR, Hodgson MJ. Blast injuries. *N Engl J Med.* 2005 Mar 31;352(13):1335–1342. doi: 10.1056/NEJMra042083. PMID: 15800229.

15. Kluger Y. Bomb explosions in acts of terrorism--detonation, wound ballistics, triage and medical concerns. *Isr Med Assoc J.* 2003 Apr;5(4):235–240. PMID: 14509125.

16. Leibovici D, Gofrit ON, Stein M, Shapira SC, Noga Y, Heruti RJ, Shemer J. Blast injuries: Bus versus open-air bombings--a comparative study of injuries in survivors of open-air versus confined-space explosions. *J Trauma.* 1996 Dec;41(6):1030–1035. doi: 10.1097/00005373-199612000-00015. PMID: 8970558.

17. Wang Z, Liu Y, Lei D, Bai Z, Zhou S. A new model of blast injury from a spherical explosive and its special wound in the maxillofacial region. *Mil Med.* 2003 Apr;168(4):330–332. PMID: 12733680.

18. Shuker ST. Maxillofacial blast injuries. *J Craniomaxillofac Surg.* 1995 Apr;23(2):91–98. doi: 10.1016/s1010-5182(05)80454-8. PMID: 7790513.

19. Stapczynski JS. Blast injuries. *Ann Emerg Med.* 1982 Dec;11(12):687–694. doi: 10.1016/s0196-0644(82)80268-0. PMID: 7149365.

20. Bagby SK. Acute management of facial burns. *Oral Maxillofac Surg Clin North Am.* 2005 Aug;17(3):267–272, vi. doi: 10.1016/j.coms.2005.05.006. PMID: 18088784.

21. Almogy G, Belzberg H, Mintz Y, Pikarsky AK, Zamir G, Rivkind AI. Suicide bombing attacks: Update and modifications to the protocol. *Ann Surg.* 2004 Mar;239(3):295–303. doi: 10.1097/01.sla.0000114014.63423.55. PMID: 15075644; PMCID: PMC1356225.

Chapter 11

Misrata and Comparative Conflicts

Abdulhakim Zaggut and Muhammad M. Rahman

Introduction

This chapter compares the types of craniofacial injuries treated in three different hospital environments:

(1) Misrata, Libya: mainly civilian injuries in a war zone.
(2) London, United Kingdom (UK): mainly road traffic accidents and some interpersonal violence.
(3) Catanzaro, Italy: mainly interpersonal violence from organised crime.

The Misrata dataset comprises of craniofacial injuries that are war related. These cases represent the greatest level of violence with the most severe injuries. In comparison, Catanzaro is similar with regards to violence-related injury involving gunshots. The London dataset is similar to that of Catanzaro as a wealth and peace environment with regards to level of medical care and availability of resources, specialists, and time afforded to a patient. The austere setting of Misrata has limited resources and, due to a high volume of casualties, less time is available for treatment and it is highly unlikely that there will be follow-up treatment. This chapter compares craniofacial injuries from an austere environment to wealth and peace settings, ultimately highlighting the importance of the craniofacial region.

A History of Contemporary Warfare

The 20th century will be remembered as one of the bloodiest with two major wars, World Wars I and II, which were fought on the European, African, and Asian continents. Since then, there have been a plethora of other wars, including the Chinese Civil War (1927–1950), the Indo–China Wars (1946–1989), three Arab–Israeli wars (1948, 1956, 1967), the Korean War (1950–1953), the Vietnam War (1955–1975) and the Iran–Iraq War (1988). The early part of the 21st century witnessed the Arab Spring uprising and subsequent dissolution in 2010–2011. In addition, there are ongoing wars at the time of writing this book, including the Syrian Civil War (since 2010), South Sudanese Civil War (2013), Central African Republic conflict (2012), Second Libyan Civil war (2014), and Second Yemeni Civil war (2015). Sophisticated and devastating arms have been used in all these hostilities, which can cause instantaneous death.

This is an observational study intended to better compare austere and war (AW) and wealth and peace (WP) in relation to injury. Austere and war is the term applied to a war zone, whereas wealth and peace has a sociological quality, both of these have unexplained origins. This chapter uses the terminology to compare the extremes of violence in three environments. These are the injuries resulting from the aggressive austere warfare in Misrata, Libya, compared to the urban WP patients admitted to the Royal London Hospital and the contrasting WP of Catanzaro in Italy.

With regards to medical treatment, in an austere environment, there are limited supplies and, with the prospect of power cuts, limited access to medical equipment. Often, large numbers of casualties can arrive and need fast treatment. In a WP environment, there is time to properly assess the injury and prepare a treatment plan with long-term follow up.

A peace setting will rarely have a major event such as a bomb blast, while this is commonplace in a war setting with war surgeons required to adapt to their austere settings to deliver life-saving treatment.

Misrata: An Austere War Setting from 2011

Misrata has an approximate population of half a million and is the third-largest city in Libya. The Arab Spring uprisings of 2010 represented a series of anti-government protests and armed civilian rebellions which swept across the Middle East in five countries. The protests originated in Tunisia, spread rapidly to Egypt, Libya, Syria, and Iraq, where civilians suffered from violence (Figures 11.1 and 11.2).

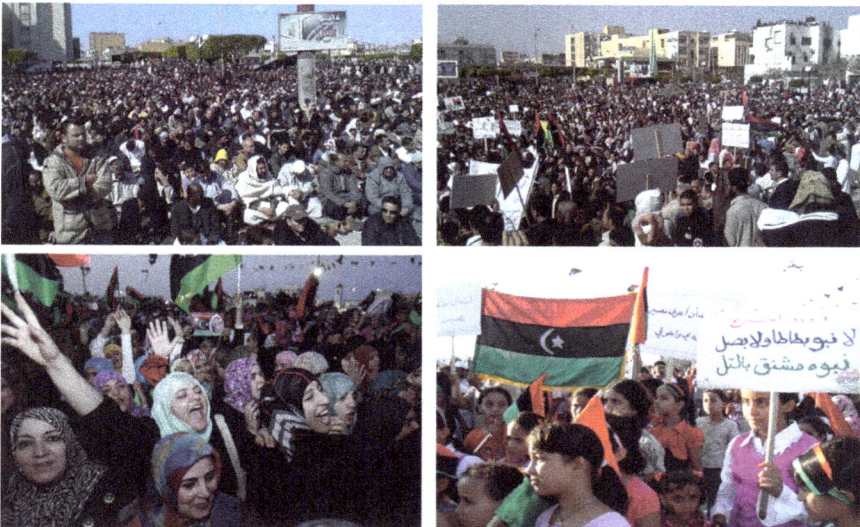

Figure 11.1   A peaceful demonstration in Misrata in 2011.

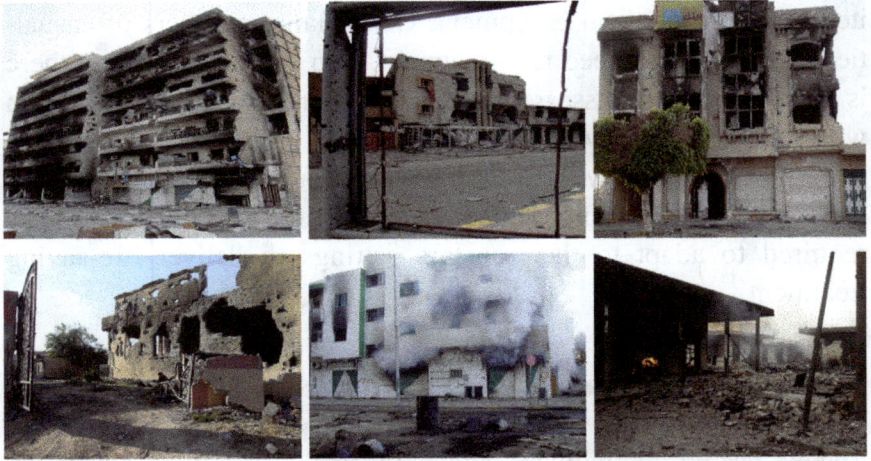

Figure 11.2   Result of Libyan civilian and government fighting.

Due to the serious shortage of experienced surgeons for the management of the Misrata wounded, a short intensive surgical course for the non-specialists was conceived and has since continued. Colonel Muammar Gaddafi governed the Libyan Arab Republic from 1969 for 42 years, but following international interventions, he was captured and assassinated in October 2011.

From 2010 to 2011, the Arab Spring uprisings spread rapidly across the Middle East, ended three dictatorships in Tunisia, Egypt, and Libya, leaving an extensive trail of destruction to civilian populations in their daily lives, as seen in the Misrata injury pattern (Table 11.1).

The Libyan civil war has continued with a power struggle involving various powers motivated by political and financial interests.[1,2] Misrata has been severely affected by a recurrent civil war from 2014 to the present with campaigns launched by four conflicting forces which have endeavoured to control the city. As a result, medical services have been overwhelmed with gunshot and blast injuries.[2,3]

The Battle of Misrata in 2011 included the occupation of the main city hospital by pro-Gaddafi forces and the targeting of city

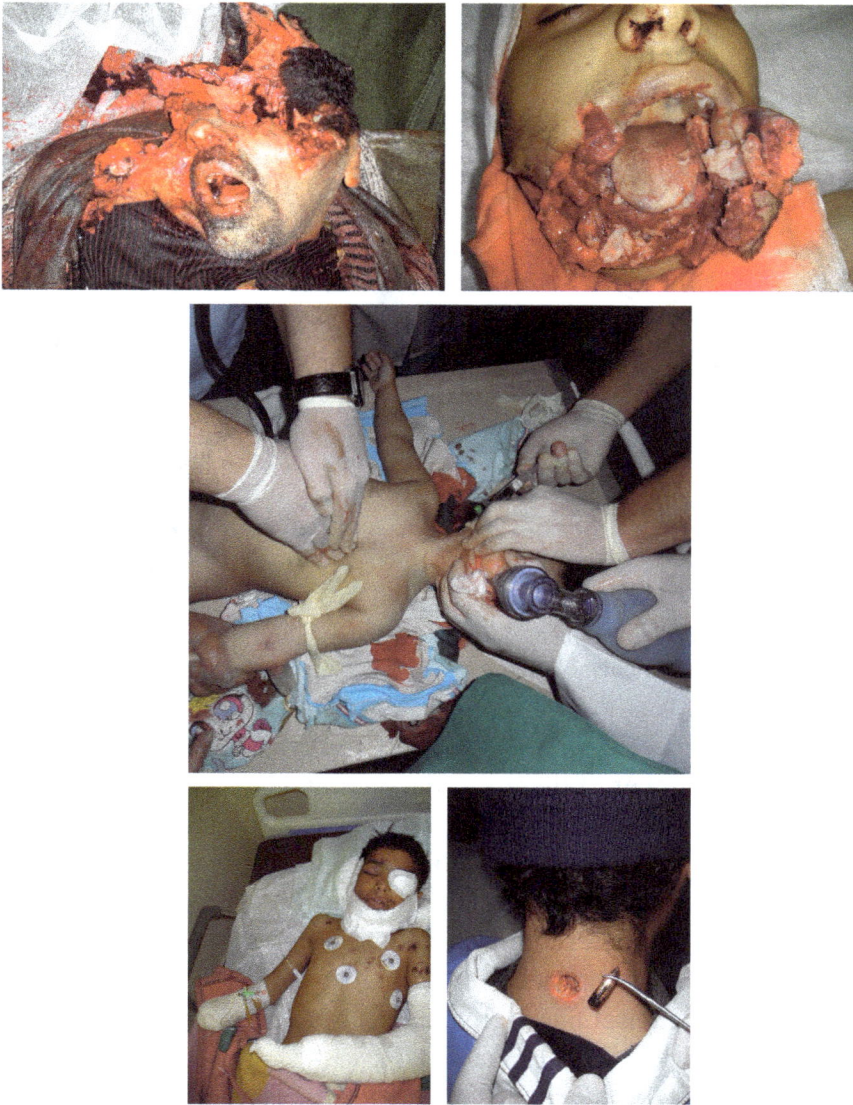

Figure 11.3 War injuries from Misrata in 2011.

polyclinics. Civilian and combatant casualties with complex injuries were treated in facilities which were ill equipped to handle such cases[4] (Figures 11.3–11.5).

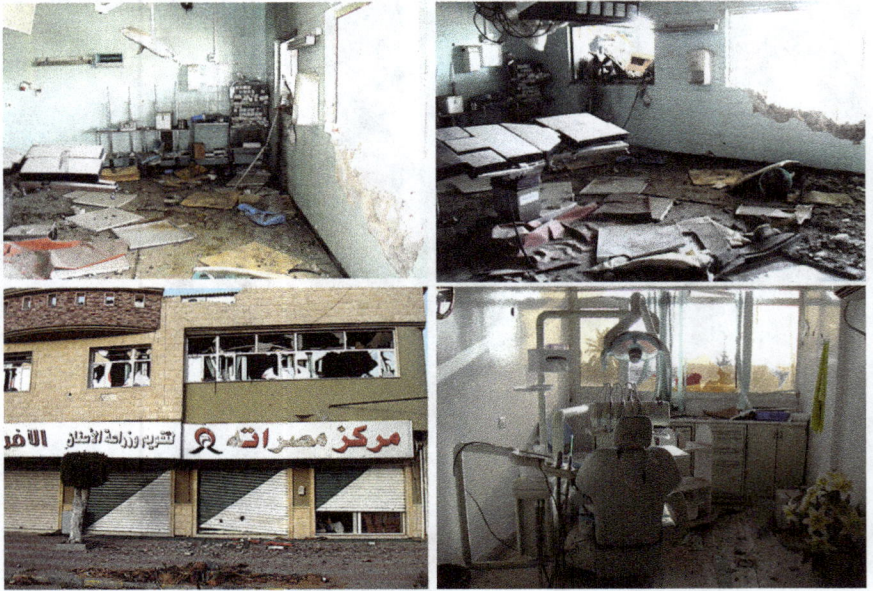

Figure 11.4 Pro-government forces targeted medical facilities by bombing hospitals, clinics, ambulance, and medical staff.

A large number of these life-threatening gunshot and blast injuries involved the head and neck region.[5] It was therefore essential that all health care providers acquired the necessary skills to achieve successful clinical outcomes. The absence of resources, severity and unpredictability of presenting cases, and lack of specialist personnel combined to create the need for specialist training.[6,7] Humanitarian emergency organisations were limited by a shortage of clinicians and supplies[2] (Figures 11.6 and 11.7).

Unfortunately, since 2011, the health service in Libya has continued to deteriorate despite the official end of the war.[8] A survey of 607 surgeons in 13 hospitals in Tripoli between June 2014 and May 2015 revealed that the hospitals were unable to deal with blast injuries and 496 surgeons (81.7%) stated that their hospitals were grossly under-equipped. Craniofacial injuries

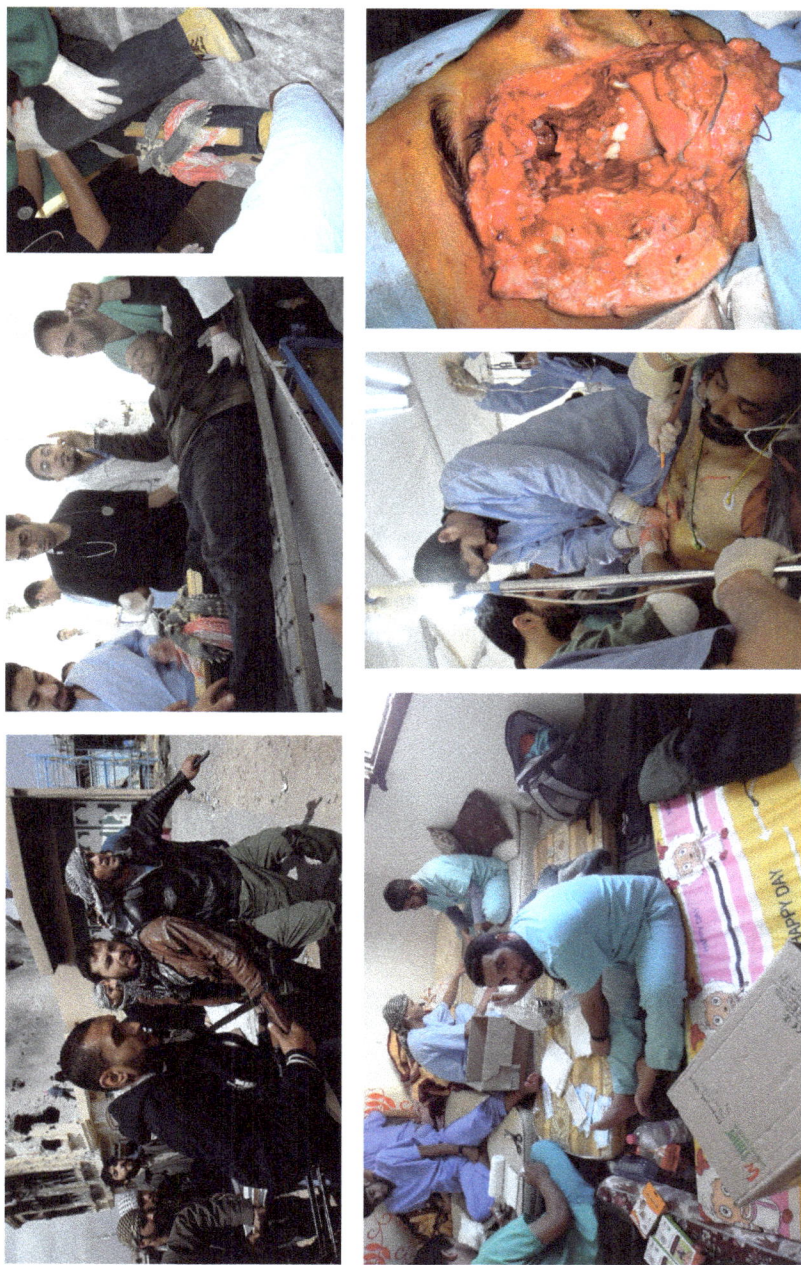

Figure 11.5 Limited resources were available to deal with life-threatening injuries.

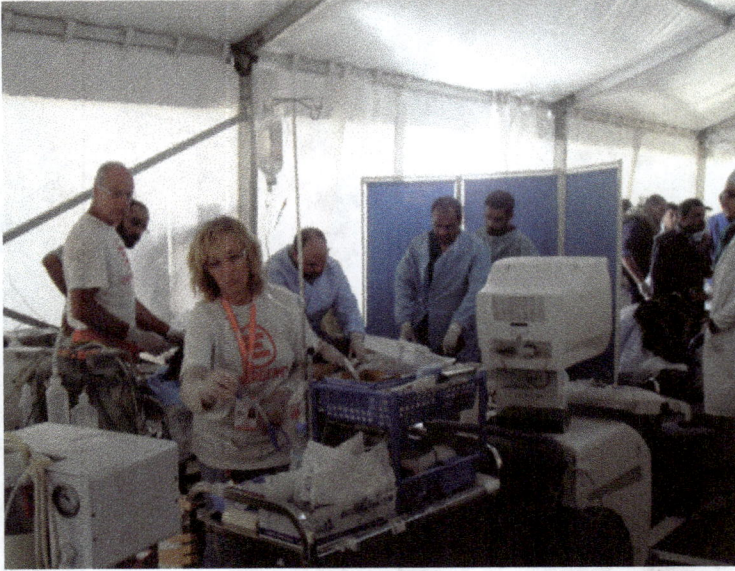

Figure 11.6   Casualties triaged and resuscitated in the corridors of Misrata Hospital due to over occupation of the emergency department space.

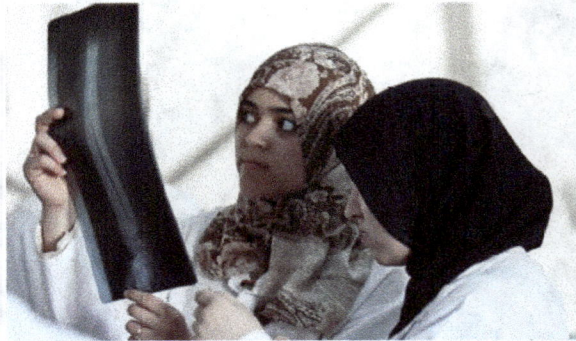

Figure 11.7   Medical students working as nurses.

represent from 20% to 39% of the total trauma burden in the major conflicts.[8–10]

As the head and neck includes the vital anatomical structures and cranial nerves, there was a need to train non-specialist professionals to become the care providers for craniofacial surgery patients (Figure 11.8). This austere environment is a unique setting with many limitations that present themselves unexpectedly. Surgery had to be performed while there were bomb blasts in close proximity which caused power cuts rendering computed tomography (CT) scanners unavailable. Having stabilised a patient's airway and controlled any haemorrhage, the next aim was to treat the craniofacial injuries. It is at this stage where training of non-specialist surgeons became invaluable.

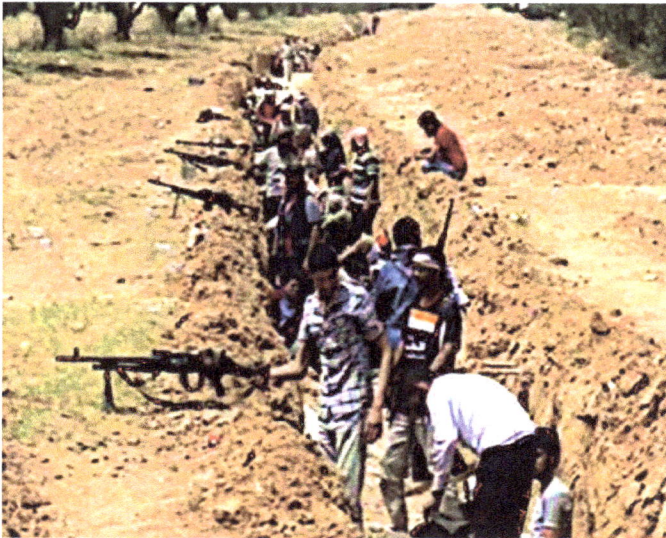

Figure 11.8 Trench warfare in Misrata in 2011. Most of the body is protected, but the head and neck area is vulnerable.

Misrata Patients and Methods

The Misrata dataset consisted of 154 craniofacial patients who were documented and treated in Misrata Hospital during the 10 months between February and November 2011. There were many undocumented cases. During these 10 months, pro-Ghaddafi troops were fighting Misrata troops and freedom fighters. Many assumed that the conflict would be concluded by Ghaddafi's death; however, fighting continues in Misrata beyond 2021.

The injury data were retrieved and analysed from the available documentation and photographs. Injuries were initially categorised into anatomical regions which included dentoalveolar injuries and fractures of the mandible, maxilla, zygoma, orbit, nasal, frontal, and cranial bones. Additional trauma sites were included, such as perioral and salivary glands, peri-orbital soft tissue and eye lids, nasal cartilage, and facial nerve injuries (Figure 11.9). The data was simplified into three broad groups: the upper face, midface including

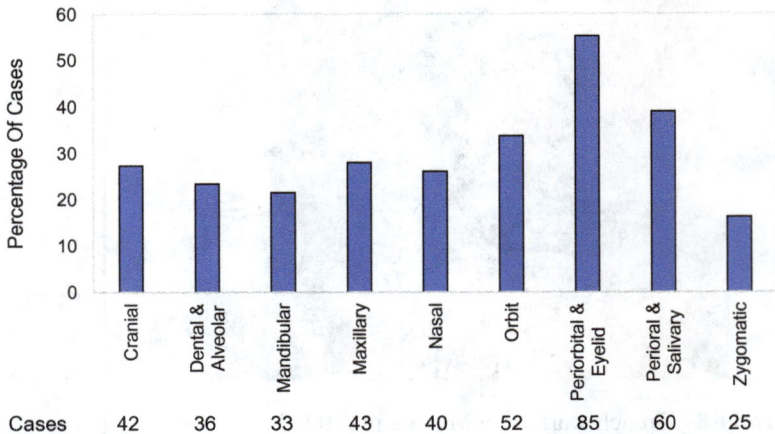

Figure 11.9   Original anatomical categories of the Misrata craniofacial injured patients.

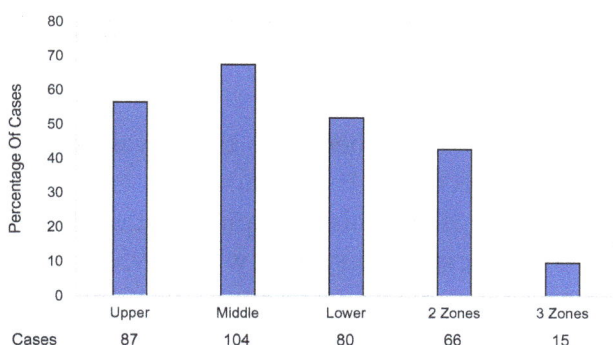

Figure 11.10 Summary of craniofacial injuries of facial thirds in Misrata.

orbit and nose, and the lower face including the oral cavity (Figure 11.10). Also recorded were those combatants who suffered injuries involving two-thirds of or entirely the face.

The majority of patients were males (146) accounting for 95% of which 83% (136) were aged between 18 and 60. There were also 16 children.

The primary causes of injury were due to blasts (75%), followed by gunshot wounds (19%). Foreign body complications involved 70% of these cases due to shrapnel or bullet wounds; however, the most common patterns of injury proved to be the five groups of facial thirds (Table 11.2).

Life-threatening injuries represent a third of the cases which included those requiring a tracheostomy or intubation in an intensive care unit or had marked haemorrhage and airway hazards due to fractured teeth. Twenty-eight (18%) of the 154 casualties suffered fatal injuries. Sixty-seven cases (43%) were classified as sight-threatening orbital injuries. Sixty-six of the total 154 cases (43%) had injuries in two areas of the face, while 15 (10%) suffered injuries to three zones. The most common form of injury was peri-orbital of which 43% were sight threatening.

Craniofacial Injuries at the Royal London Hospital in East London

The second dataset was obtained from the Royal London Hospital (RLH) based in Whitechapel, East London.

This is the principal teaching hospital in East London, which has a major maxillofacial surgery unit, where 593 craniofacial cases during the year 2012 and 717 cases during 2013 were treated. The cohort consists of 1,310 consecutive cases, in which 5% of cranial injuries were referred for neurosurgery. As with the Misrata data, these injuries were classified into facial thirds.

Interpersonal violence targeted the lower facial third (54%), followed by the middle third which included the nose and orbit (40%) and finally the upper facial third (11%). Most patients sustained craniofacial injuries to one facial third (90%), whereas involvement of all three facial areas was rare (1%). In contrast to Misrata, less than 1% injuries were caused by gunshots and none were blast injuries.

Catanzaro: An Urban Wealth and Peace Setting (2006–2016)

A third dataset was collected from Catanzaro, an Italian city of 91,000 inhabitants, which is the capital of the Calabria region (Figure 11.11).

This cohort consisted of 35 civilian patients with craniofacial injuries treated at the University Hospital (Università degli Studi Magna Graecia) in the 10 years between 2006 and 2016.

Here, the trauma was interpersonal violence from organised crime. The injuries were Mafia-related, consisting of assault, gunshot, and blast injuries as well as knife wounds. The data collected were provided by Professor Amerigo Ghudice, an oral and maxillofacial surgeon. These 35 cases in a WP zone in southern Italy were

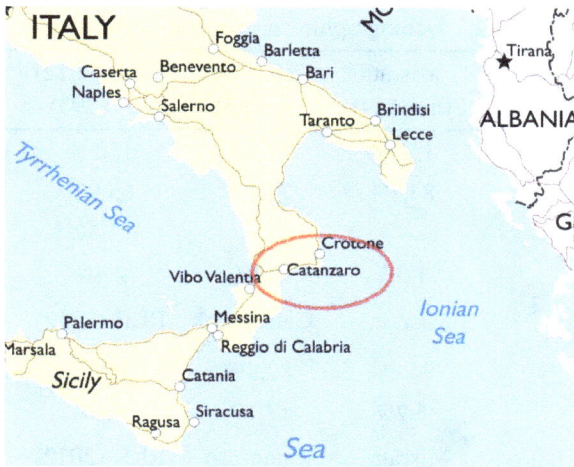

Figure 11.11   Catanzaro, South Italy is an urban WP setting.

used to compare with the AW trauma cases in Misrata and the urban WP trauma cases of the Royal London Hospital.

Results

On comparing the three datasets, the commonalities between these are the age and gender of patients. Misrata had the greatest number of blasts and gunshots followed by Catanzaro (Table 11.1). London injuries consisted of interpersonal assaults. As expected, foreign bodies were only found in Misrata patients.

All datasets showed similar percentages of injuries to the middle and lower thirds of the face and significantly more injuries to the upper third in Misrata patients, likely to be the result of blast injuries (Table 11.2). For this reason, there was a large percentage of injuries to two facial thirds in the Misrata patients while ~90% of the Catanzaro and London injuries only affected one facial third. This also correlates with injury severity in Misrata cases (Table 11.3).

Table 11.1 Demographic comparison of the datasets.

Age Group	Misrata (*n* = 154)	Catanzaro (*n* = 35)	RLH (2012) (*n* = 593)	RLH (2013) (*n* = 717)
<18	15.6%	17.1%	18.5%	14%
19 – 40	83.1%	77.1%	65.9%	68.1%
41 – 60			13.3%	16.9%
>60	1.3%	5.7%	2.4%	1%
Gender	Misrata	Catanzaro	RLH (2012)	RLH (2013)
Male	94.8%	82.9%	86.3%	93.2%
Female	5.2%	17.1%	6.6%	6.8%
Mechanism of injury	Misrata	Catanzaro	RLH (2012)	RLH (2013)
Interpersonal assault	0%	0%	35.2%	28.5%
Blasts	75.3%	14.3%	0%	0%
Gunshot	19.5%	25.7%	0.3%	0.4%
RTA	3.9%	N/A	N/A	N/A
Other	1.3%	0%	0%	0%
Foreign bodies	Misrata	Catanzaro	RLH (2012)	RLH (2013)
Shrapnel	78%	NIL	NIL	NIL
Bullet wounds	22%	NIL	NIL	NIL

Table 11.2 Summary of craniofacial injuries by facial 'thirds'.

Injury by Facial thirds	Percentage of Cases (%)		
	Misrata (*n* = 154)	RLH (2012) (*n* = 593)	RLH (2013) (*n* = 717)
Upper third	56.5	10.9	7.7
Middle third	67.5	46	51.2
Lower third	52	54	51.2
One third	47.4	90	90.3
Two thirds	42.9	8.1	10.1
Three thirds	9.7	1.4	0

Table 11.3 Craniofacial cases classified by severity.

Injury Severity	Percentage of Cases (%)	
	Misrata ($n = 154$)	Catanzaro ($n = 35$)
Life-threatening	33	23
Sight-threatening	44	31
Soft tissue	73	40
Nerve injury	67	46

Discussion

There has been a change in modern war where hostile human violence is taking place in urban areas and not just on the battlefield, notably in civilian-targeted terrorist attacks which have been carried out in both highly urbanised and traditional rural settings.[11] Patients with craniofacial injuries treated in AW zones have no access to expert services and are often treated by non-expert health care providers.[5] To optimise patient care in these circumstances, it is necessary to identify the knowledge base and competencies that can be safely taught to non-specialist providers. The literature on medical education has insufficient information about what educational intervention can be used to address the increasingly escalating global issue of violent human conflict in non-battlefield areas.

Craniofacial injuries are increasing: terrorist attacks and wars in civilian communities are becoming more common.[9] The effect of violent human conflict on the health services has resulted in the general consensus that such events present unusual and difficult challenges for any civilian health care provider to deal with.[11] The literature indicates a lack of knowledge as well as a lack of basic surgical skills for treating craniofacial injuries in relation to the competencies of non-specialists. Indeed, one health care provider during his duty of treating war injuries questioned: 'Are we to blame for our insufficient performance or was there something else?'. Treating war injuries can present a major challenge for junior doctors and even surgeons with extensive experience in accident and emergency, who feel their performance is inadequate when confronted with complications arising from violent human conflict.[7] Current surgical training curriculums for both undergraduates and postgraduates are relatively poor in covering the management of craniofacial injuries.[12,13] In this context, Elledge and McAleer reported that accident and emergency staff in the UK lack confidence to deal with common maxillofacial trauma.[8] As a result, health care providers should be familiar with trauma from austere environments such as blast injuries.[14] It is therefore important to enhance the surgical training standard through implementation of an appropriate training program that will optimise the service outcome, in particular enhance patient results and change the fundamental knowledge base of the non-specialist.

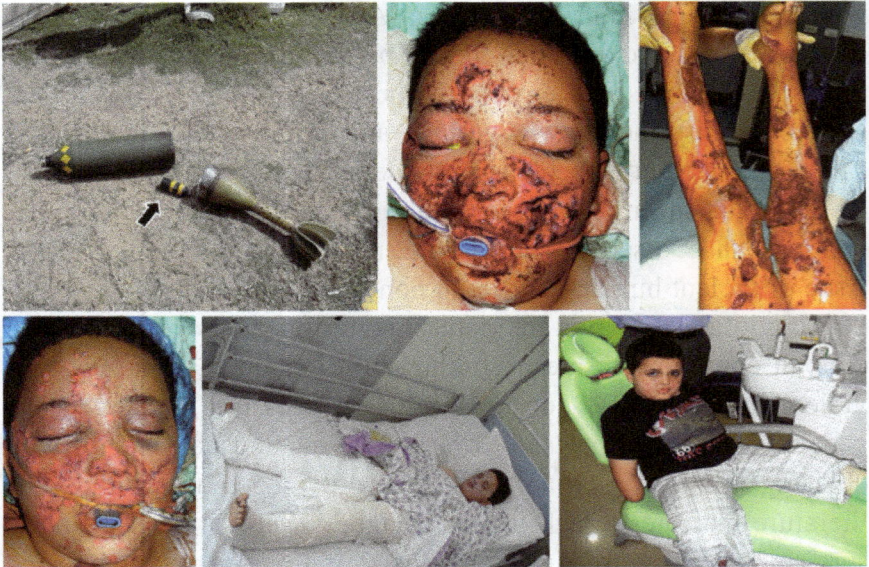

Figure 11.12   Eight-year-old child amputee after handling a cluster bomb in Misrata.

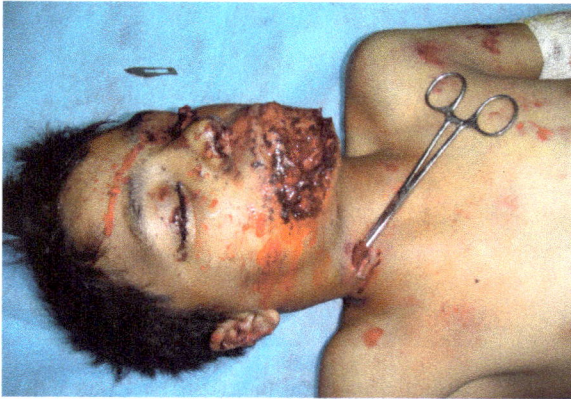

Figure 11.13 Eleven-year-old child amputee with left eye perforation after handling a cluster bomb in Misrata.

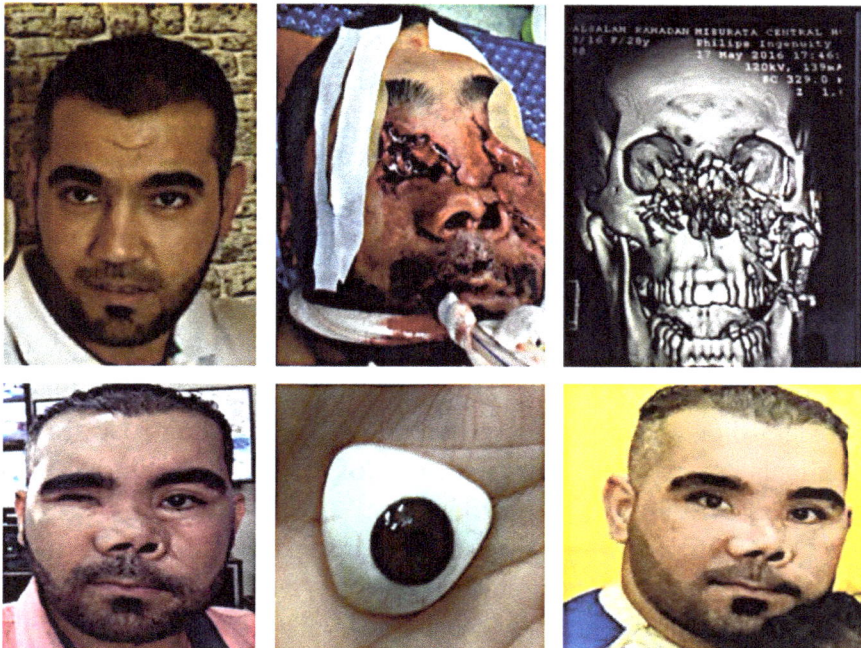

Figure 11.14 Islamic State militant (ISM) terrorist in 2016 with a midface blast injury. The upper-left frame is prior to the injury. The adjacent clinical photograph and 3-D CT scan show right orbit and nasion comminution. The mid-lower row shows the right prosthetic eye and result of surgery.

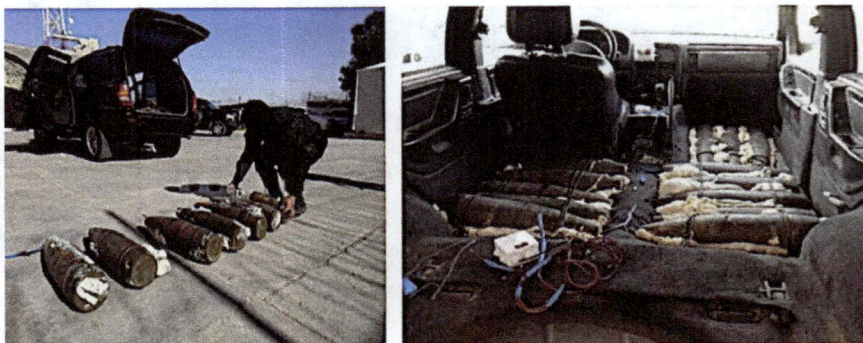

Figure 11.15   Islamic State militant (ISM) car bomb in Libya.

Unlike Catanzaro and London, military weapons with large destructive range, such as cluster bombs which inflict multiple injuries within seconds, are commonly used[15] (Figures 11.12–11.15).

Although the Catanzaro data are qualitative, there is a major disparity in numbers over the 10 years. The qualitative features are the results of interpersonal violence which involved aggressive weapons and knives, all characteristic of organised crime.

However, the Misrata data which was collected in 10 months provides insight into the pattern of craniofacial injuries during a bloody civil war.

As anticipated, the majority of patients were aged between 18 and 60 years and the cause of most injuries were explosive blasts with gunshot wounds ranking second, both exceeding road traffic accidents which is the primary cause of craniofacial injuries in a non-war environment, such as London.

The severity of war injuries has progressed over time with traditional armaments being replaced by explosive bombs and bullets. Craniofacial injuries are now caused by high-velocity blasts leading to severe destruction of both soft and hard tissues with foreign bodies in the wounds, further complicated by infection. Furthermore, there were increased numbers of sight-threatening injuries, although

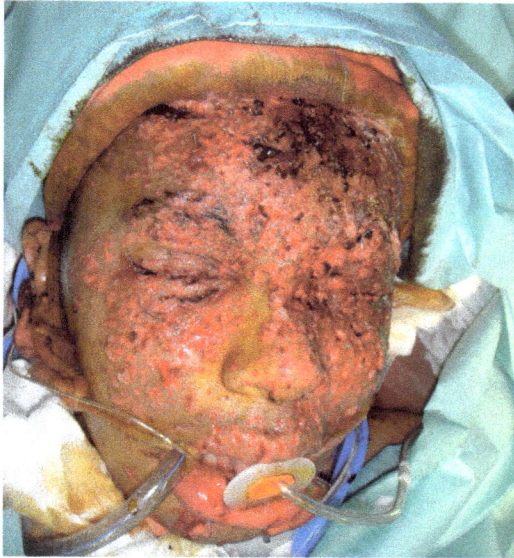

Figure 11.16   Blast injury causing complete loss of sight and multiple facial wounds post cleaning from impregnated with debris, rocks, and sand.

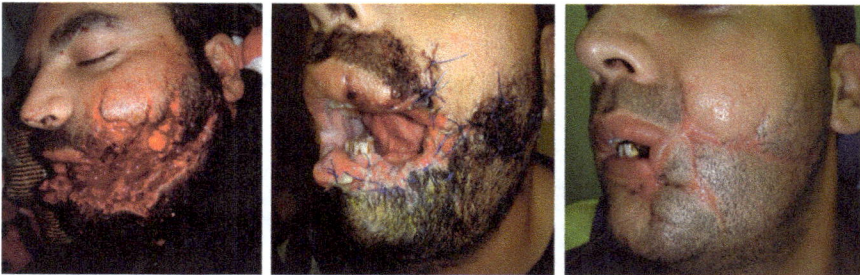

Figure 11.17   Cheek and facial lacerations. Male victim sustained facial soft-tissue injury one year post operation.

these may be fewer than first thought due to concomitant fatality. Clinical examples of Misrata war injuries are given in the following (Figures 11.16–11.21).

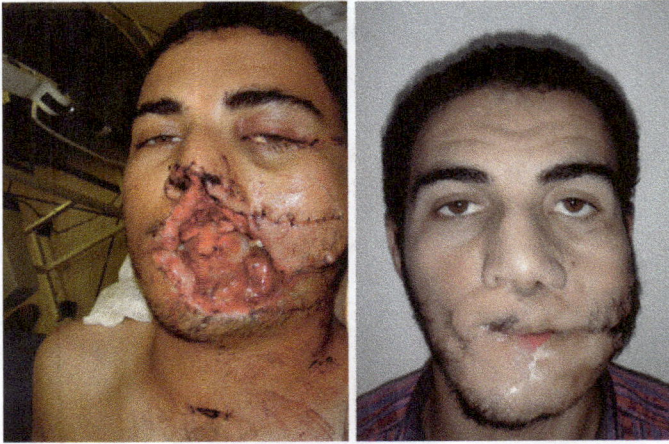

Figure 11.18   Civilian war injury denoting the severity and complexity of craniofacial war trauma.

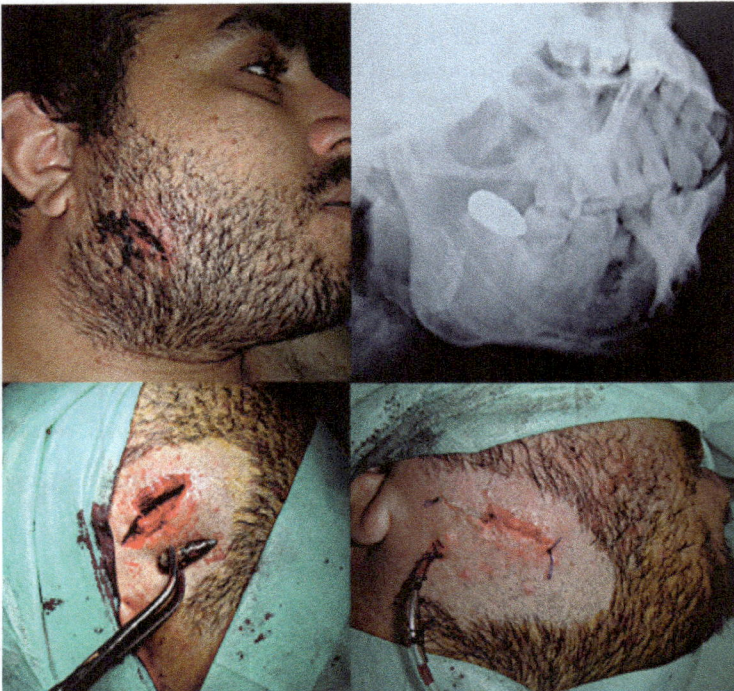

Figure 11.19   Gunshot wound to the right mandible and the removed bullet.

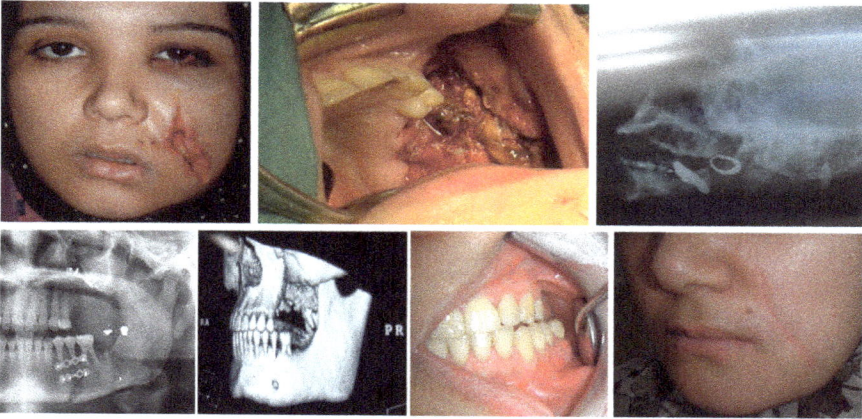

Figure 11.20   Foreign body (shrapnel) penetration of the maxillofacial region.

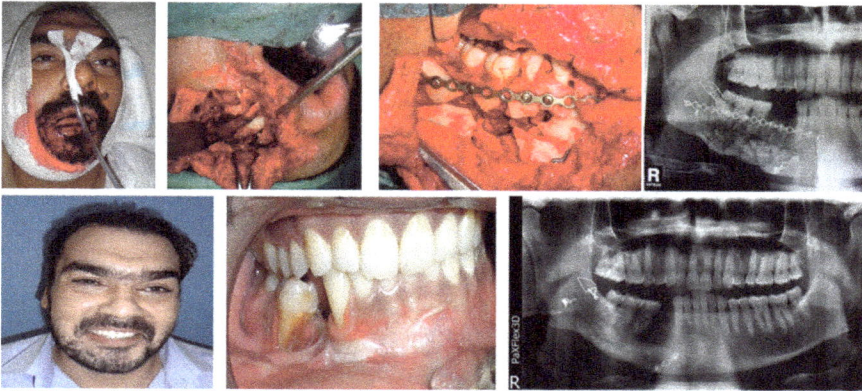

Figure 11.21   Comminuted mandibular fractures with avulsion of hard and soft tissues, open reduction with internal fixation during initial surgery.

The warfare data from Misrata shows that the middle third of the face was most affected with 104 facial thirds out of the 154 combatants. Two facial thirds were involved in 66 cases. This appeared to be an index of violence in a war zone as well as the lack of protection of the mid facial area.

Unfortunately, the inability to apply a standardised quantification or classification systems, such as the ZS system which is available on smart phones, restricted the data analysis. The absence of prior training on the care of war victims impaired the documentation analysis as many of the surgeons lacked experience of an AW and chaotic environment. Follow-up appointments to review the patients would have provided a better indication of outcome.

Conclusions

The comparison of the three datasets shows that blast and gunshot injuries from military-grade weapons dictate the severity of injury. This also implies that if such weapons were used in WP environments, there would be a similar severity to craniofacial injuries. It is apparent that AW and WP are socio-economic terms and not an accurate demographic classification of conflict. A WP setting may describe the RLH in Whitechapel but does not accurately represent the terrorism incidents that occurred elsewhere in Birmingham, Manchester, or Paris with regards to injury type. These studies provide a guide for the development of strategies to prevent craniofacial injuries in all aggressive environments. This is especially important due to the random nature of terrorist attacks that can occur in high-population areas where blast and bullet associated injuries are rare.

Despite the tragedy of war and conflicts worldwide, there have been valuable surgical management techniques practiced and developed during times of violent human conflict. Surgeons in the conflict zones are desperate for surgical support to save lives, and craniofacial surgeons are in great demand in these situations.

The data presented in this chapter are documented in the author's PhD thesis, available online at *bit.ly/wartrauma:*

Design & validation of a simulation training course for the management of acute Craniomaxillofacial (CMF) austere & war trauma by non-specialists.

References

1. Albira IA, *et al.* Post-war waste composition: Household waste management in Misrata City, Libya. *Arab World Geogr.* 2018;21(2–3):114–127.
2. Kuperman AJ. Obama's Libya debacle: How a well-meaning intervention ended in failure. *Foreign Aff.* 2015;94:66.
3. Review WP. Libya population 2019. 2019 May 12. http://worldpopulation review.com/countries/libya-population/.
4. Ng C, *et al.* The Libyan civil conflict: Selected case series of orthopaedic trauma managed in Malta in 2014. *Scand J Trauma Resusc Emerg Med.* 2015;23:103.
5. Esmil T, *et al.* Management of casualties in Misrata following the civil uprising in Libya, with an emphasis on maxillofacial injuries. *Fac Dent J.* 2015;7(1):40–45.
6. Zaggut AW, Rahman MM, Youssef G, Holmes S, Ellamushi H, Shibu M, Ghanem A, Myers S, Harris M. Craniomaxillofacial war injuries in Misrata, Libya. *J Dent.* 2020 Aug.
7. Zaalook K. Whom shall we save when at war? A personal perspective on the Libyan conflict. *Afr J Emergency Med.* 2013;3(1):40–41.
8. Oun AM, Hadida EM, Stewart C. Assessment of the knowledge of blast injuries management among physicians working in Tripoli Hospitals (Libya). *Prehosp Disaster Med.* 2017;32(3):311–316. doi:10.1017/S1049023X17000127.
9. Lew TA, *et al.* Characterization of craniomaxillofacial battle injuries sustained by United States service members in the current conflicts of Iraq and Afghanistan. *J Oral Maxillofac Surg.* 2010;68(1):3–7.
10. Wade AL, *et al.* Head, face, and neck injuries during operation Iraqi freedom II: Results from the US navy-marine corps combat trauma registry. *J Trauma Acute Care Surg.* 2007;63(4):836–840.
11. Gataa IS, Muassa QH. Patterns of maxillofacial injuries caused by terrorist attacks in Iraq: Retrospective study. *Int J Oral Maxillofacial Surg.* 2011;40(1):65–70.
12. Clayton R, Perera R, Burge S. Defining the dermatological content of the undergraduate medical curriculum: A modified Delphi study. *Br J Dermatol.* 2006;155(1):137–144.
13. Elledge RO, McAleer S. Planning the content of a brief educational course in maxillofacial emergencies for staff in accident and emergency

departments: A modified Delphi study. *Br J Oral Maxillofac Surg.* 2015;53(2):109–113.

14. DePalma RG, *et al.* Blast injuries. *N Engl J Med.* 2005;352(13):1335–1342.
15. Reuters. This is what the inside of an ISIS car bomb looks like. 2018 [cited 2021].https://globalnews.ca/news/3959498/this-is-what-the-inside-of-an-isis-car-bomb-looks-like/.

Chapter 12

Civilian Gunshot Injuries in Pakistan

*Saad Uddin Siddiqui, Muhammed Aqeel Aslam and
Syed Mahmood Haider, with Hajra Rana and
Zia Uddin A. Kashmiri*

Introduction

Projectile weapons originate from ancient times. After the invention of gunpowder in the 12th century, weapons progressed to cannons, guns, and tanks. Later, the spread of ammunition-based weapons extended to many societies and increased the incidence of ballistic injuries in the civilian population. Projectile weapons have been responsible for high morbidity and mortality ever since. The craniofacial region is often left unprotected by armour, and it is also a common target for suicide attempts and interpersonal violence.

Understanding a Gunshot Wound

It is imperative to understand the characteristics of firearm injuries in order to diagnose and treat them.

Figure 12.1 shows the two types of gunshot projectiles found in civilian gunshot wounds. One is the bullet form, which has a metal

217

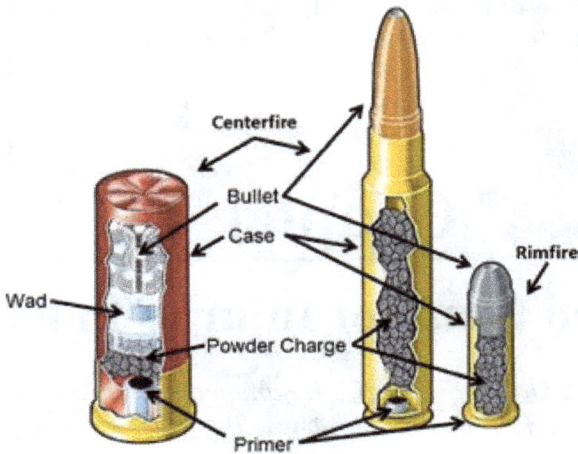

Figure 12.1   Shotgun and bullet cartridges.

jacket composed of brass or copper and causes penetrating injuries. The shape of the bullet determines its piercing potential; however, penetration into the tissues is determined by its momentum which depends on its size, weight, and velocity. A pointed bullet which is large and heavy has more penetration potential than a round-tipped, small light bullet (Figure 12.2).

The weapons which fire bullets include rifles that have long barrels while pistols or revolvers have short barrels. Damage to the deep tissues should be expected owing to the high penetration potential of the bullet. Another type of gunshot projectile is the multiple pellets of a shotgun cartridge, which spread upon firing and cover a wider area. The pellets have less penetration capacity and are mainly responsible for a widespread avulsive type of injury.[1]

Classification of Gunshot Injuries

The closer the source of the projectile, the greater the injury. Gunshot wounds can be classified according to the range of fire:

(a) Contact injury: The weapon is held against the body.
(b) Short-range injury: The weapon is held within six inches (15 cm).

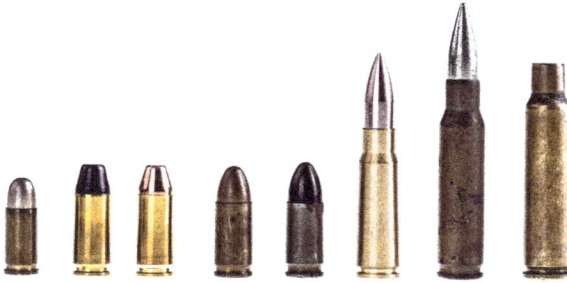

Figure 12.2   Various sizes and shapes of bullet.

(c) Intermediate-range injury: The weapon is held between 6 and 36 inches (15–90 cm).

(d) Long-range injury: The weapon is held further than 36 inches (90 cm).

The kinetic energy of the projectile is another important factor in determining the extent of the injury. The projectile causes a tearing and crushing injury to the soft and hard tissues because of its inertia. Hard tissues suffer comminution, and the resultant small fragments act as secondary projectiles transmitting the kinetic energy to the adjacent soft tissues, leading to further shearing and avulsive injuries.

KE = ½m(v₁–v₂)²

$$KE = \tfrac{1}{2}m(v_1 - v_2)^2$$

- **KE** is the kinetic energy, measured in joules (J);
- **m** is the mass of the projectile (e.g. the bullet);
- v_1 and v_2 are the velocities at entry and exit, respectively.

Based on their kinetic energy, gunshot wounds can be classified as low energy (100–500 J) and high energy (up to 3000 J).

Another classification is by speed:

- Low velocity: less than 1,200 ft/s ($\approx$366 m/s).
- Medium velocity: 1,200–2,000 ft/s.
- High velocity: greater than 2,000 ft/s ($\approx$610 m/s).

Entry and Exit Wounds

The size of the entry wound in a bullet injury is similar to the diameter of the bullet (Figure 12.3). Depending on the density of the tissues, the trajectory of the missile can change due to bullet deflection and drag. The bullet may be stopped by tissue resistance and remain embedded in the body, in which case its location can be determined by radiography or scanning.

However, with high-velocity injuries where the bullet exits the body, the exit wound is typically larger than the entrance wound. The entry and exit wounds reveal the path of the bullet inside the body and the tissues encountered during its course.

Injury from a shotgun at close range produces particles and gases, creates a blast-like pattern, and the penetration of the pellets is less than that of a bullet. Injuries caused by shotgun fire are wide and avulsive with significant tissue damage at the entry site but not necessarily as deep as those from a high-velocity bullet.

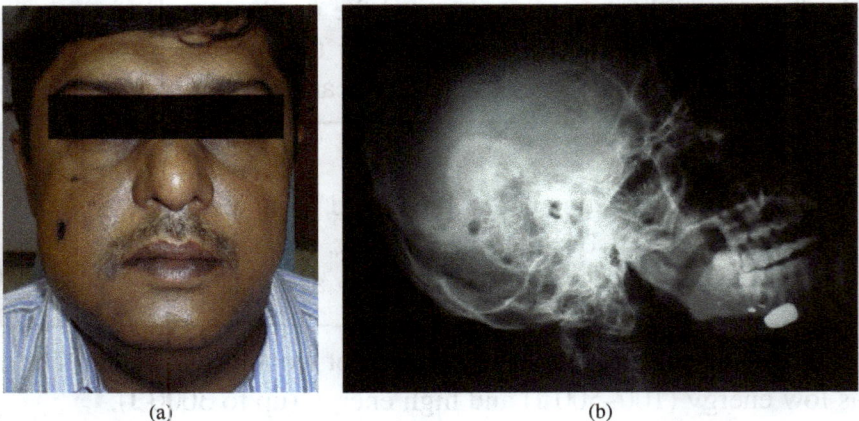

(a)   (b)

Figure 12.3   (a) Entry wound at the right cheek. Note that the size of this entry wound is the same diameter as the bullet shown in Figure 12.4(b); (b) Due to its low energy and low velocity, the bullet was arrested in the right buccal sulcus.

In Figure 12.4, the size of the entry wound is large and cavern-ous with significant tissue loss, but the patient's airway is patent signifying low-penetrating injury. The radiograph shows a shattered angle of the mandible on the left side. In an austere environment, clinicians often have to work with poor-quality images like this (see Chapter 7). Here, the retained pellets are barely visible.

Nerve Injuries

Gunshot wounds to nerves rarely transect the nerve and usually cre-ate a stretch or compression injury along the bullet trajectory. Small-calibre, low-velocity civilian gunshot wounds may lead to a partial nerve injury with only some loss of function. High-velocity hunting or military gunshot injuries produce more devastating loss of tissue and neurologic function.

Unless immediate surgery is required for a neurological deficit, the patient is observed and scanning studies are performed three weeks after the incident. A lack of recovery by three months should prompt surgical exploration. If the nerve has been completely tran-sected, primary repair or a graft is performed. Intraoperative nerve

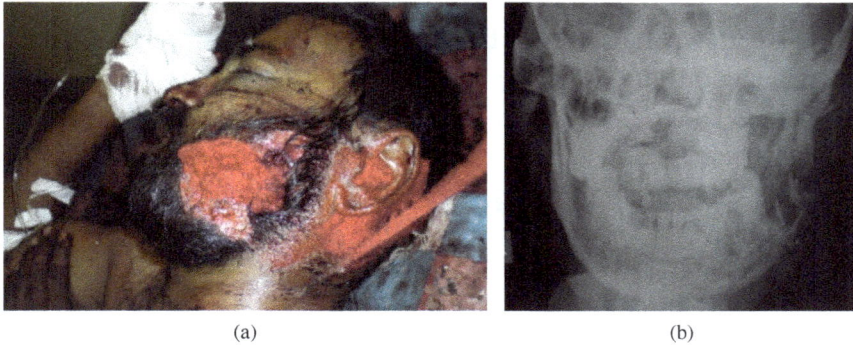

(a)   (b)

Figure 12.4 (a) Short-range and high-velocity shotgun wound; (b) Radiograph of the patient.

action potential recordings are used to evaluate nerve lesions in continuity, and those that show no conduction are treated by resection and grafting.

Two-thirds of nerve suture repairs and about half of the nerve grafts show a meaningful clinical improvement. Delayed intervention and long grafts suffer the worst outcomes.

(For more details about facial nerves, see Chapters 3 and 4.)

Management of Gunshot Wounds

As shown, gunshot wounds vary from minimal abrasion to devastating tissue loss.

The injury is caused primarily by the projectile and secondarily by the target fragments hitting the adjacent tissue.

The management of gunshot injuries can be divided into the following phases:

(a) Resuscitation and stabilisation.
(b) Reconstruction.
(c) Rehabilitation.

Resuscitation and Stabilisation

The primary management of ballistic craniofacial injury relies on the advanced trauma life support (ATLS) protocol, as discussed in detail in Chapter 2. The key concerns are the airway, achieving haemostasis, and cervical spine management, then to identify bone fractures and foreign bodies, splint fractured bone segments, and other injuries.

Airway Control

Nearly one-half of patients with facial ballistic injuries have a compromised airway due to injury of the upper respiratory tract.[2] Oral endotracheal intubation is the preferred method to maintain the airway as nasal intubation is not recommended in cases of middle or upper third facial injuries. Establishing a surgical airway, such as a cricothyroidotomy, may be warranted in cases of excessive orofacial tissue laceration, bleeding, or laryngeal injury.[3]

A fibre-optic intubation technique can be helpful to secure the airway in the absence of blood and vomit (aspiration may be necessary) but requires specialist equipment and an experienced anaesthetist. If the severity of the maxillofacial injury suggests the need for prolonged intubation, an early elective tracheostomy must be considered.

Haemorrhage

Facial gunshot injuries can be complicated by significant blood loss due to the vascularity of the head and neck. Bleeding from blasted tissues requires pressure and immediate gauze packing. Closure of the wound helps to achieve haemostasis in up to 90% of patients (Figure 12.5).

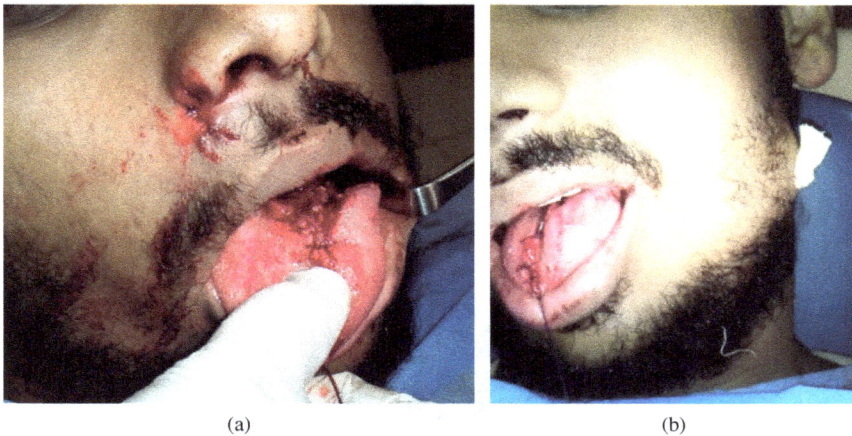

(a) (b)

Figure 12.5 (a) Entry wound at the right nostril with the bullet's pathway lacerating the tongue; (b) Exit below the left ear. Closure of the tongue laceration achieved haemostasis.

Anterior and posterior nasal packing are effective means to control haemorrhage from the maxillary sinus and nose, as shown in Figure 12.6.

Bleeding from major vessels may warrant electrocauterisation, ligation, or embolisation via angiography. Using a Foley catheter may help to achieve haemostasis, as described in Chapter 1.

Suction enables the surgeon to identify and ligate, clamp, or cauterise the bleeding vessels. Blind clamping is to be avoided because adjacent vessels, nerves, or other important structures may be damaged. As perfusion of the head and neck is mainly through branches of the external carotid artery, ligation of the external carotid artery is considered when other techniques fail. Blood should be cross matched in cases of excessive bleeding, in which case a blood transfusion needs to be arranged.

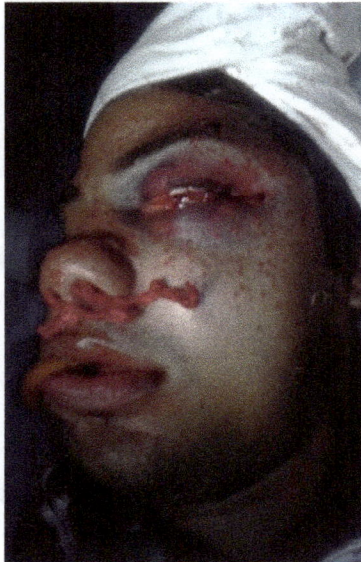

Figure 12.6   Anterior nasal gauze packing applied to arrest the bleeding from the nose.

Posterior epistaxis is defined as active bleeding despite adequate anterior packing or when no bleeding point is identified by anterior rhinoscopy. Bleeding points are identified by rigid nasal endoscopy for cautery. As the first line of treatment, endoscopic diathermy or arterial ligation is effective and should be used where available. Unfortunately, the expertise and apparatus to perform this are not yet available universally.[4,5]

Posterior nasal packing with a Foley catheter is an effective and rapid non-surgical alternative in the management of posterior epistaxis (see Chapter 1). This is commonly performed in conjunction with anterior packing using either nasal tampons or ribbon gauze lubricated with Vaseline or bismuth iodoform paraffin paste.

Fractured segments of facial skeleton cause bleeding and shearing injuries to soft tissues. The splinting and stabilisation of these fractured bony segments using stainless-steel wires helps in achieving haemostasis, conserving the bone for future reconstruction and providing framework for initial soft-tissue closure, as shown in Figure 12.7.

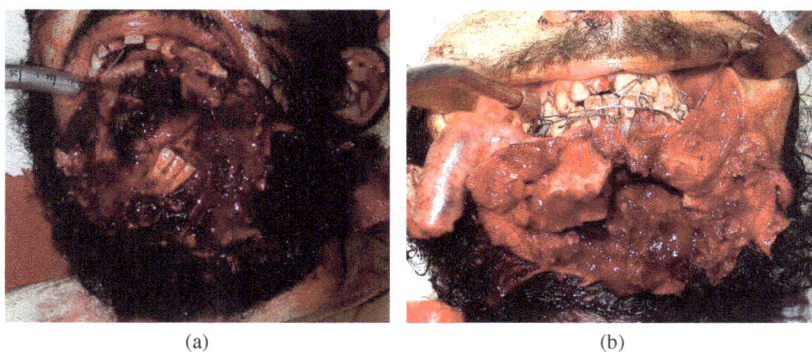

(a)　　　　　　　　　　　　　(b)

Figure 12.7 (a) Grossly comminuted fractured segments of the mandible with shearing injuries and bleeding into the soft tissues; (b) Splinting and stabilisation of the fractured bone segments with stainless-steel wire to achieve haemostasis, conserving the bone for reconstruction and providing a framework for soft-tissue closure.

Overall management for gunshot injuries is as follows (Figures 12.8–12.10):

- A head-to-toe examination is mandatory.
- A low Glasgow coma scale may indicate a concomitant brain injury.

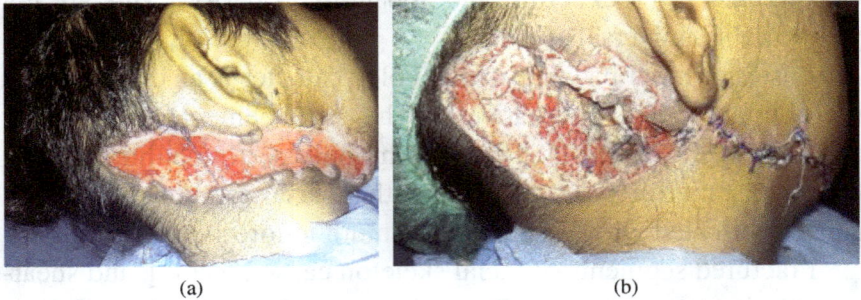

Figure 12.8   (a) Skin loss due to a gunshot wound; (b) Delayed management of necrosis due to thermal injury and infection resulting in further loss of tissue.

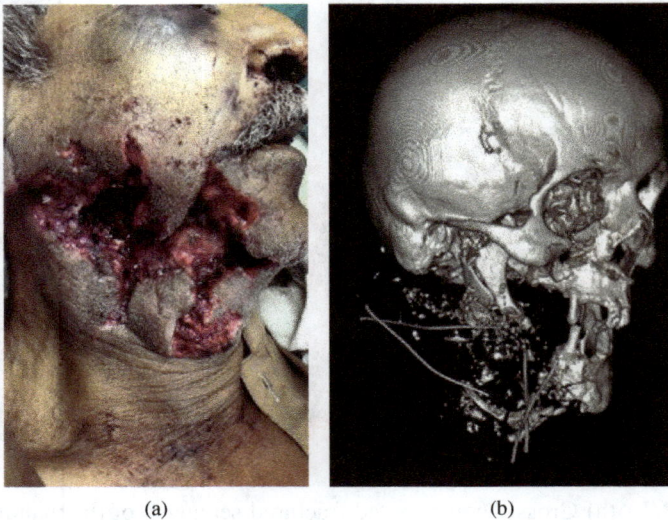

Figure 12.9   (a) Contaminated close-range shot gun wound with major tissue loss of the right face overlying the mandible but below the eye and nose; (b) computed tomography (CT) scan showing the extensive destruction of the right facial skeleton.

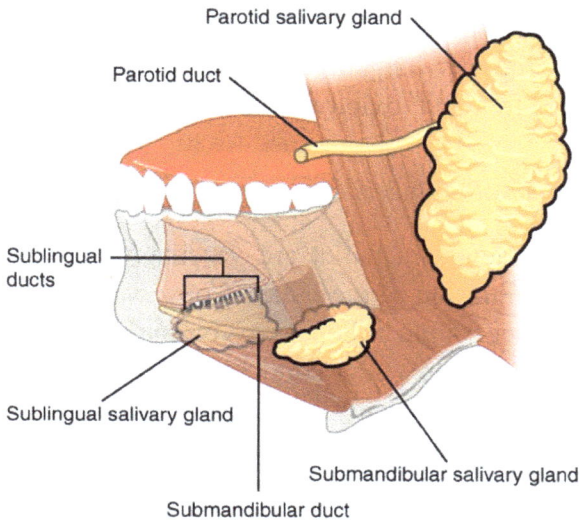

Figure 12.10   Diagram showing the complex of salivary glands and their ducts damaged by a blast resulting in salivary fistulae.

Source: Image licensed under CC BY-SA 3.0. By Connexions, OpenStax College, Anatomy & Physiology, Connexions Website. http://cnx.org/content/col11496/1.6/, June 19, 2013.

- Cervical spine precautions must always be established and cleared by both clinical and radiographical examination.
- Injuries to the brain, thorax, abdomen, or other areas of the body necessitate the involvement of other specialists.
- Negative pressure of blast air results in the penetration of contaminated debris into the deeper tissues. Although the empirical use of broad-spectrum antibiotics is believed to increase the prevalence of bacterial resistance, broad-spectrum antibiotics should be used to treat both Gram-positive and Gram-negative bacteria. This delays the time and expense that would be required to perform definitive culture and sensitivity.
- Gross contamination also necessitates tetanus prophylaxis.
- Retrieval of bullet and pellets is not a mandatory part of this phase, although superficial pellets and debris can be removed with caution.

• A significant amount of lead is found in firearm projectiles; therefore, copious irrigation of the tissues with warm clean water helps to avoid toxicity.

Retrieval or Removal of Bullets

The risks of retrieving a bullet are vascular injury, nerve injury, infection, and migration of the bullet. Conservative management is proposed for inaccessible bullets in asymptomatic patients to avoid iatrogenic injury (Figures 12.11 and 12.12).

Removal surgery is only planned when the bullet can be extracted safely without risk to adjacent structures. The position of the bullet must be accurately established before the procedure. Retrieval can be done either percutaneously or endoscopically; endoscopic retrieval can be guided with ultrasound and CT scan. When extracting a bullet embedded in soft tissue, it is important to avoid bullet migration. To prevent this slippage, a figure-of-eight

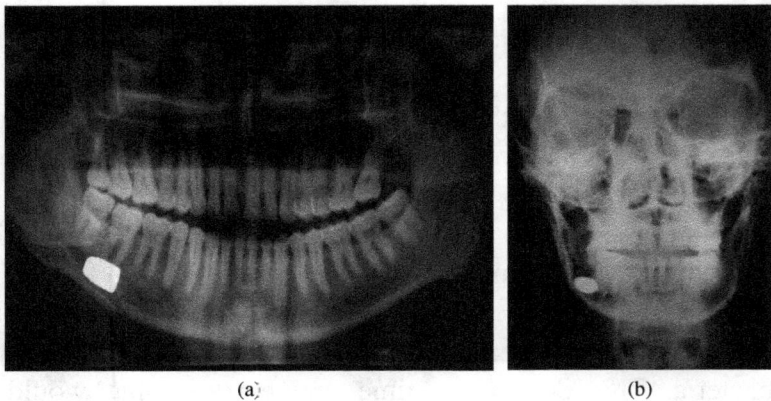

(a)   (b)

Figure 12.11   (a) and (b) Intermediate-velocity bullet causing a monocortical fracture of the mandible and trapped inside the mandibular body. The patient had no paraesthesia and the teeth were vital, hence the bullet was left in place to avoid the risk of iatrogenic damage.

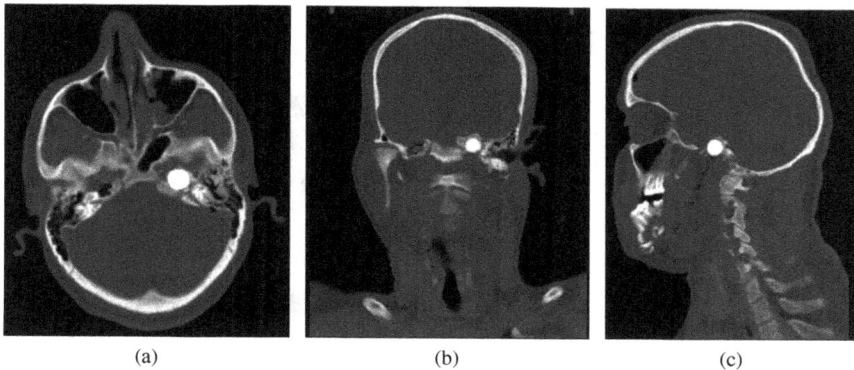

(a)   (b)   (c)

Figure 12.12 (a–c) Inaccessible bullet embedded in the base of the skull. Retrieval was not attempted due to risk of brain and cranial nerve damage.

suture or simple digital retention should be made proximal to the bullet site while manipulating it.

Figure 12.13 demonstrates how a palpable superficial bullet was retrieved through a percutaneous approach under local anaesthesia. The incision was made parallel to the branches of the facial nerve to avoid facial nerve paralysis or weakness.

Reconstruction Phase

Reconstruction of ballistic head and neck injuries is challenging and requires restoration of a substantial number of structures and their function. Soft-tissue defects need skin cover and oral lining, achieved by closure or grafts.

The surgeon may have to achieve wound closure where the tissue is not just separated but torn away from the underlying fractured facial bones. This must be explored carefully, prior to initiation of any reconstruction.

Appropriate imaging is necessary to clearly identify the extent of the fractured segments and the presence of foreign bodies. CT

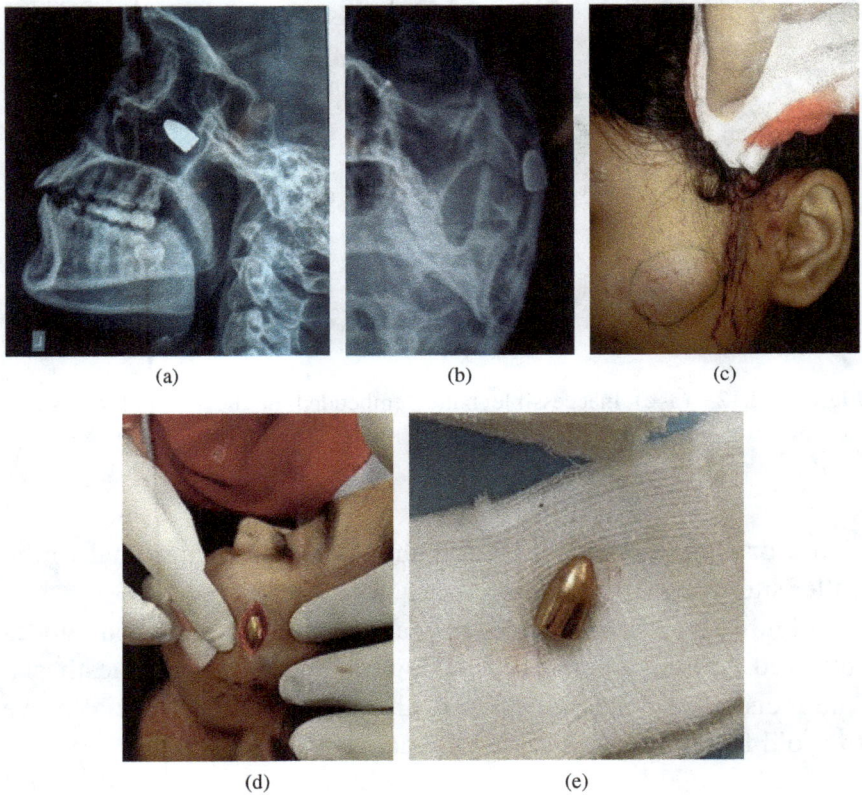

(a)   (b)   (c)

(d)   (e)

Figure 12.13   (a–e) Retrievable bullet in the subcutaneous maxillary area.

with 1-mm slices and three-dimensional reconstruction images is the study of choice to obtain accurate information while keeping a stable cervical spine. An orthopantomogram (OPG) is also needed to assess the dentition and jaws.

Local soft-tissue flaps are desirable for facial reconstruction due to their appropriate colour and texture. However, in cases of significant tissue loss, a regional or distant flap is necessary. A variety of such flaps have been utilised for reconstruction in the head and neck region. These include the temporalis, deltopectoral, pectoralis major, latissimus dorsi, and free vascularised flaps.

Jaw fracture segments can be corrected either with closed reduction and intermaxillary fixation or open reduction and intermaxillary fixation with miniature plates and screws.

The closed reduction preserves viable bone fragments and prevents any compromise of periosteal blood supply. However, a closed reduction does not always result in anatomical correction and requires more time to heal and achieve normal function. Healing can also be compromised by soft-tissue entrapment between bone fragments resulting in non-union.

By contrast, open reduction with internal fixation has the advantage of approximating fractures under direct vision. This results in anatomical restoration, optimum fixation, and early return to function.[6] Open reduction is also essential for reconstruction of continuity of bone cortices by grafting in cases of severe comminution and bone loss.

Figure 12.14 shows the reconstructive phase in a gunshot injury to the mandible.

Stereolithographic models are an advanced means of accurately planning skeletal reconstruction of a comminuted facial skeleton, as used in the reconstruction in Figure 12.15.

When there is discontinuity of the mandible, the tongue can be prevented from falling back at the time of extubation by suturing it to a mandibular reconstruction plate.

Rehabilitation Phase

Rehabilitation procedures are intended to increase functional activity, correct any obvious reconstructive errors and improve the cosmetic appearance of the patient.

Common procedures performed during this phase include adjustment of eye, ear, and dental implants.

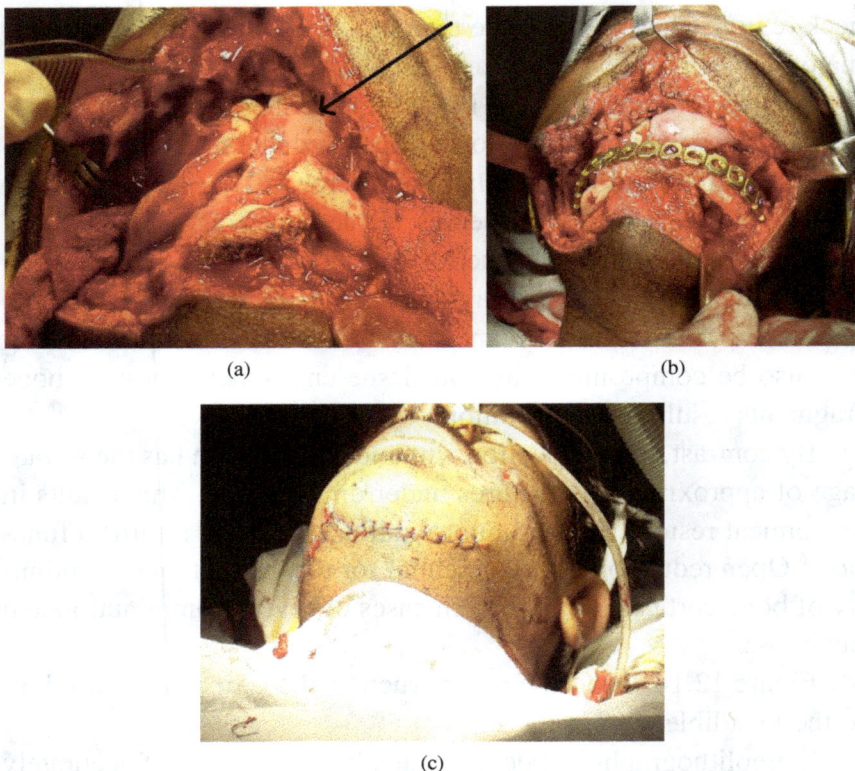

Figure 12.14   (a) Tongue protruding between the comminuted fractured man-dibular bone remnants; (b) Open reduction and internal fixation using a mandibu-lar reconstruction plate to retain a bone graft. The tongue rests on the bone gap and can be anchored temporally to the fixation plate; (c) After closure of the laceration.

Other considerations include pre-prosthetic procedures, such as vestibuloplasty and ridge augmentation, or orthognathic surgery to correct maxillary-mandibular arch discrepancies.

Scar contractures and damage to the temporomandibular joint may limit facial movement and physical therapy in the form of a mouth stretching device, such as the TheraBite, can be useful (Figure 12.16). However, stretching scar tissue presents a great challenge due to contracture and may require a flap replacement.

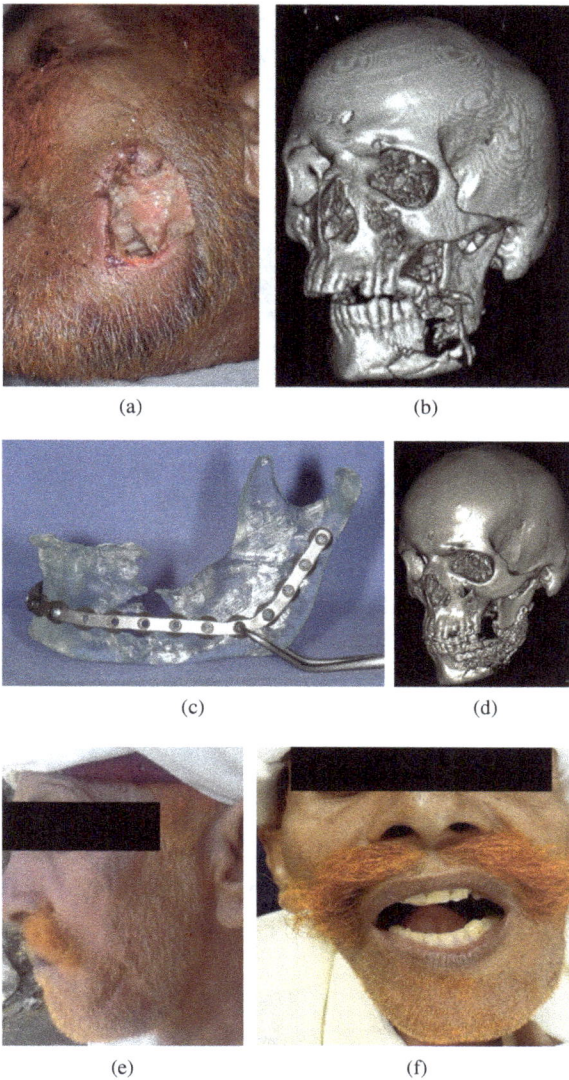

(a)　　　　　　　　　　(b)

(c)　　　　　　　　　　(d)

(e)　　　　　　　　　　(f)

Figure 12.15　(a) Facial soft-tissue defect overlying the comminuted fracture of the left angle of the mandible with bone loss; (b) CT scan showing the major bone loss in the left body and angle of the mandible; (c) 3-D stereolithographic model reconstruction of a comminuted fractured mandible enables a precise reconstruction; (d) 3-D CT bone scan showing the accurate open reduction and internal fixation with a bone graft and reconstruction plate; (e) and (f) Six months post-operative.

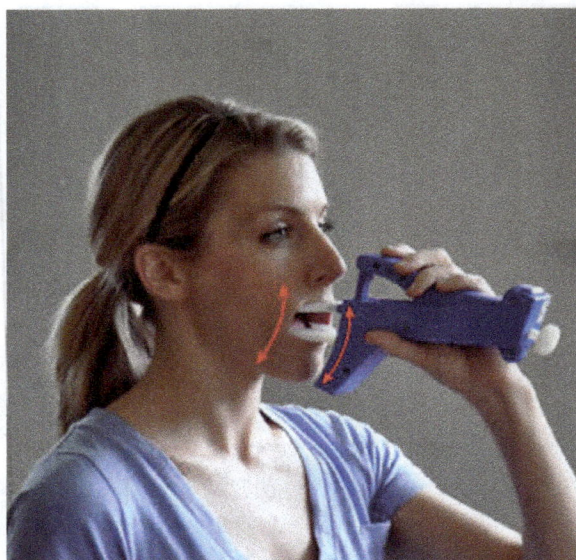

Figure 12.16   Using a TheraBite to extend the opening of an extra-articular ankylosed mandible to overcome a contracture.

A Case Study

In 2010, a patient suffered a left facial gunshot wound with the loss of his left eye and creation of a palatal fistula.

The Management Phase (Figure 12.17)

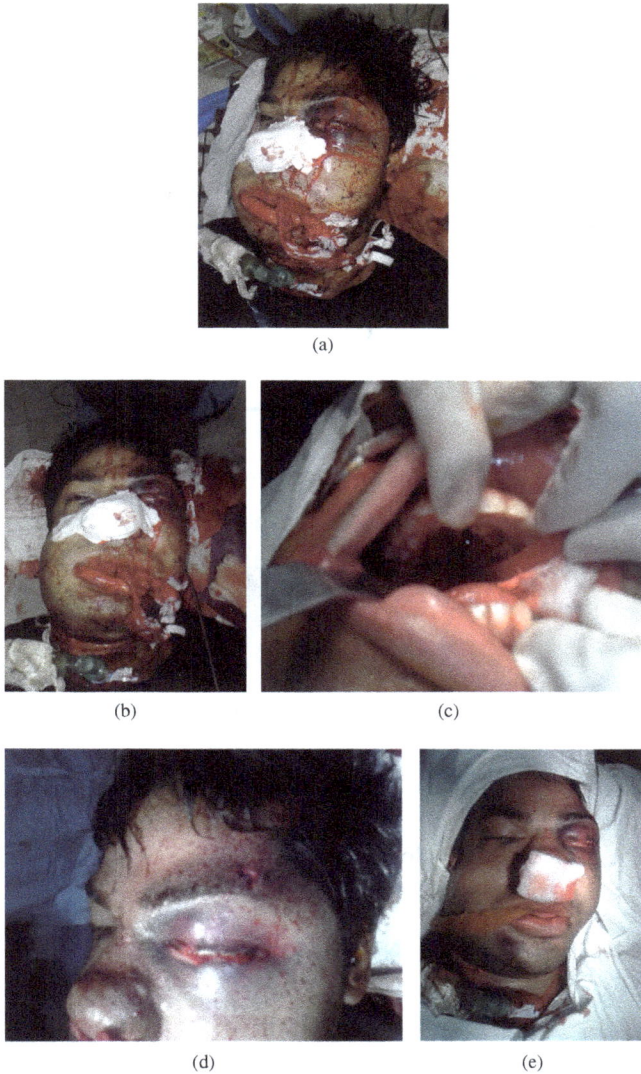

Figure 12.17 (a) Bullet through the left palate, tongue, and mandible. The airway is established with a tracheostomy due to excessive bleeding; (b–e) Phase 1 management: Entry wound at left supraorbital area and smaller exit wound at right submandibular region. High-velocity bullet causes fracture of left supraorbital rim, perforation of left eye, hard palate, shearing of lateral tongue, and fracture of right mandibular body.

The Reconstruction Phase (Figure 12.18)

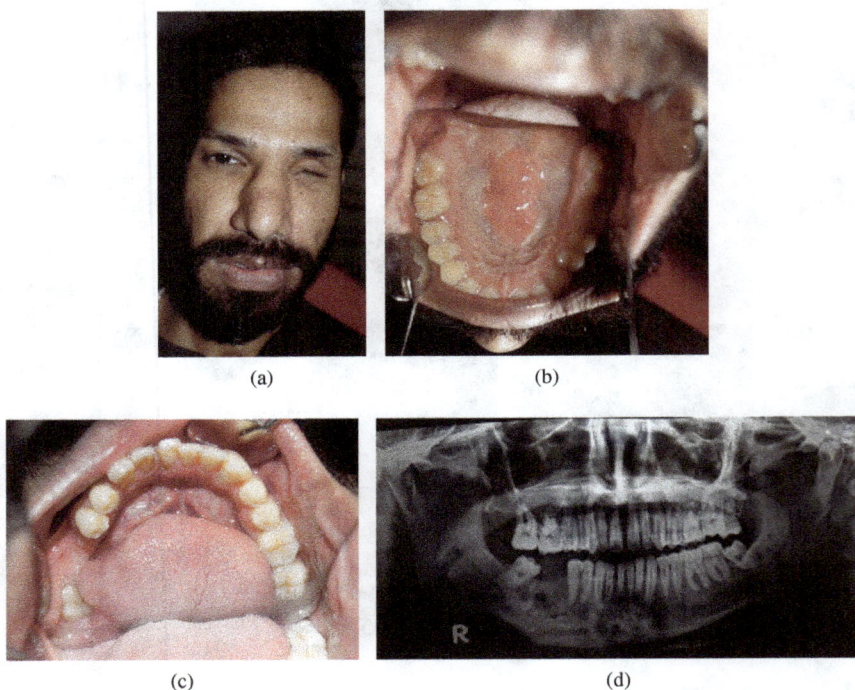

(a)   (b)

(c)   (d)

Figure 12.18 (a) Same patient 10 years later; (b) Palatal fistula has been recon-structed with a buccal mucosal flap; (c) and (d) Healed fracture of the right man-dibular body using IMF and closed reduction. The patient has paraesthesia of lower lip due to inferior alveolar nerve injury.

The Rehabilitation Phase (Figures 12.19-12.21)

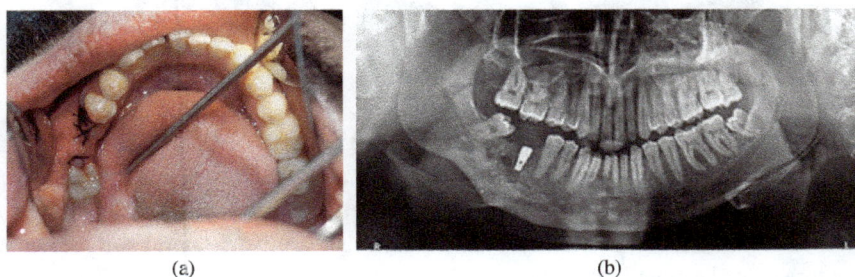

(a)   (b)

Figure 12.19 (a) and (b) Dental implant placed in lower-right first molar area providing successful dental rehabilitation.

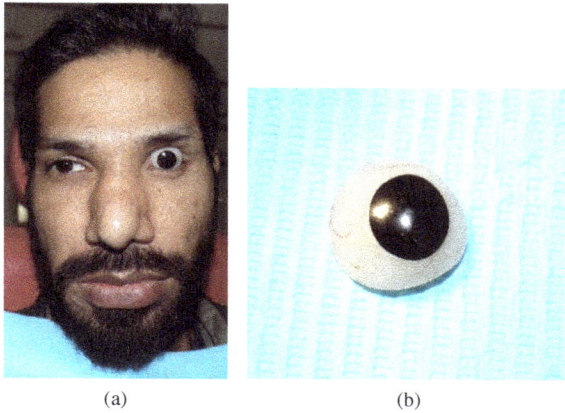

Figure 12.20 (a) and (b) Patient's eye implant was extruded due to its mismatch with orbital scarring which required revision surgery to enable it to fit.

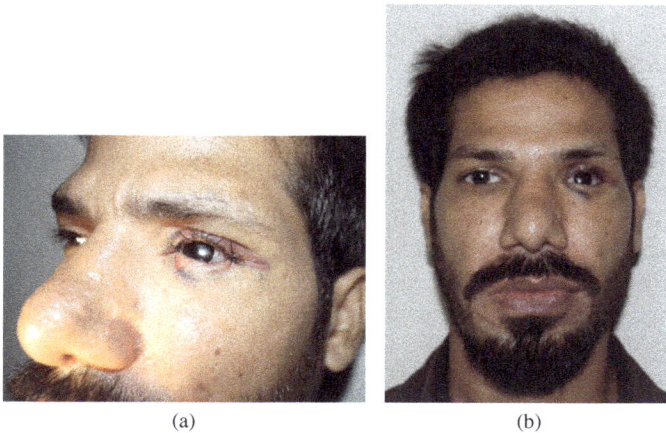

Figure 12.21 (a) and (b) Immediately post operative and one week post operative.

Conclusion

Gunshot wounds to the craniofacial area can cause many long-term problems for the patient. There are multiple considerations given the high probability that a number of factors will need to be addressed, not solely the bullet wound. The extraction of the bullet is the primary concern, but there are various checks that are required to ensure that there is no nerve damage, loss of sight, or mechanical damage to the jaw. After this, aesthetics are the next consideration. From the perspective of war zone, the immediate need is to save the patient, but the surgeon also knows that there are unlikely to be follow-up appointments, in which case the patient's quality of life and long-term health can be significantly improved with certain procedures (see Chapter 1) and any aesthetic improvements should also be prioritised.

References

1. Amir H, Dorafshar ED. Management of avulsive gunshot wounds to the face. In: Bagheri SC (Ed.), *Current Therapy in Oral and Maxillofacial Surgery*, (St. Louis, Missouri, Elsevier Saunders, 2012), pp. 361–365.
2. Bukhari SG. Management of facial gunshot wounds. *J Coll Physicians Surgeons Pak.* 2010;20(6):382–385.
3. Glapa M, Kourie JF, Doll D, Degiannis E. Early management of gunshot injuries to the face in civilian practice. *World J Surg.* 2007;31(11):2104–2110. doi:10.1007/s00268-007-9220-2.
4. John Breeze NM. Management of military ballistic injuries to the face and neck. In: Brennan PA (Ed.), *Maxillofacial Surgery*, 3rd Ed, (St. Louis, Missouri, Elsevier, 2017), pp. 230–242.
5. Lin BR. Gunshot wounds. In: al PT (Ed.), *Ferraro's Fundamentals of Maxillofacial Surgery*, (New York, Springer, 2015), pp. 257–264.
6. Saad-Ud-Din Siddiqui. Efficacy of open reduction and internal fixation in achieving bony union of comminuted mandibular fractures caused by civilian gunshot injuries. *The Surgeon.* 2020 Aug;18(4):214–218.

Chapter 13

Civilian Gunshot Injuries in Arizona, USA

Sabah Kalamchi

Introduction

Ballistic facial trauma is common in the United States (US), including mass shootings which are for the most part an American phenomenon. Firearm injury is the second leading cause of death after road traffic accidents, with an annual mortality of approximately 33,000.

Furthermore, 19,000 suicides represent 66% of these gun deaths. In addition, there are around 12,000 homicides, approximately 750 cases from unintentional shootings (2%) with approximately 300 ballistic deaths from police intervention and 250 cases of undetermined intent.[1] This has directly resulted in the development of the US Level 1 well-equipped trauma hospitals.

Six Craniofacial Ballistic Injuries Showing the Difficulties of Reconstruction

The following examples of high-energy ballistic facial injuries illustrate the significant challenge of facial reconstruction.

The terms used to classify these wound injuries are **high-velocity wounds** (faster than 2000 ft/s ≈ 610 m/s) and **low velocity** for lesser speeds.

However, these criteria do not necessarily translate into distinct clinical injuries, and more useful terms are **avulsive** and **nonavulsive** injuries.

Avulsion is where a body structure is torn off, and the term is most commonly applied to surface trauma where all layers of the skin have been lost leaving the underlying structures exposed.

Nonavulsive injuries, such as fractures, tend to be comminuted with the majority of the soft tissue remaining intact. The fracture can usually be treated by closed management with repair of the overlying laceration.

The avulsive facial injuries, which result from high energy transfer with varying degrees of soft tissue and bone loss, pose a particular reconstructive challenge. These avulsive injuries generally result from a shotgun at close range, a rifle, or a high-powered handgun. As we will show in this chapter, these avulsive injuries require a soft-tissue envelope to be reconstructed over the skeleton within two weeks of the injury to avoid irreversible scar contracture.

Case 1

A 51-year-old female was brought to Scottsdale Healthcare Centre with a self-inflicted gunshot wound to the face after a suicide attempt (Figure 13.1). The patient was immediately intubated and transported to the trauma centre intensive care unit (ICU).

The computed tomography (CT) scans showed right orbital fractures, and within 24 hours, she was taken for surgery, including open reduction with fixation of the left orbital fractures and repair of the overlying facial wound.

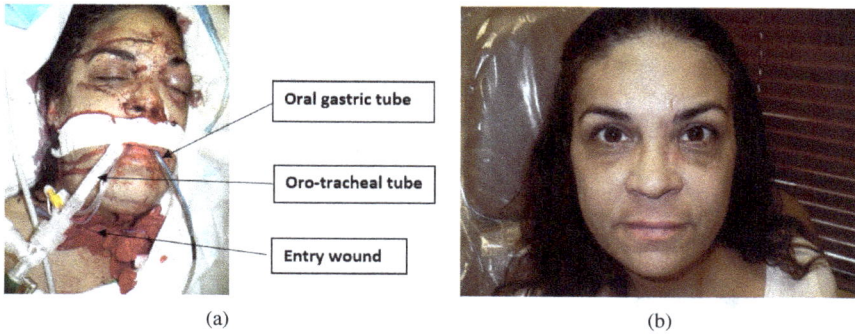

Figure 13.1 Case 1: (a) A 51-year-old female with a single gunshot wound to the chin, on a ventilator with an orotracheal tube; (b) Three months post injury.

Case 2

A 74-year-old male attempted suicide with a gunshot to the chin. He was intubated in the trauma bay at Scottsdale Healthcare trauma centre. The CT scan shows an edentulous mandible with comminuted fractures but minimum clinical soft-tissue damage (Figure 13.2).

The patient was operated on the following day to the injury when the oral endotracheal tube was changed to a naso-endotracheal tube. The edentulous patient underwent internal and external reduction and fixation of the mandibular fractures.

The mandibular fracture was treated with a mandibular internal plate and external pin fixation. The lip laceration was also sutured.

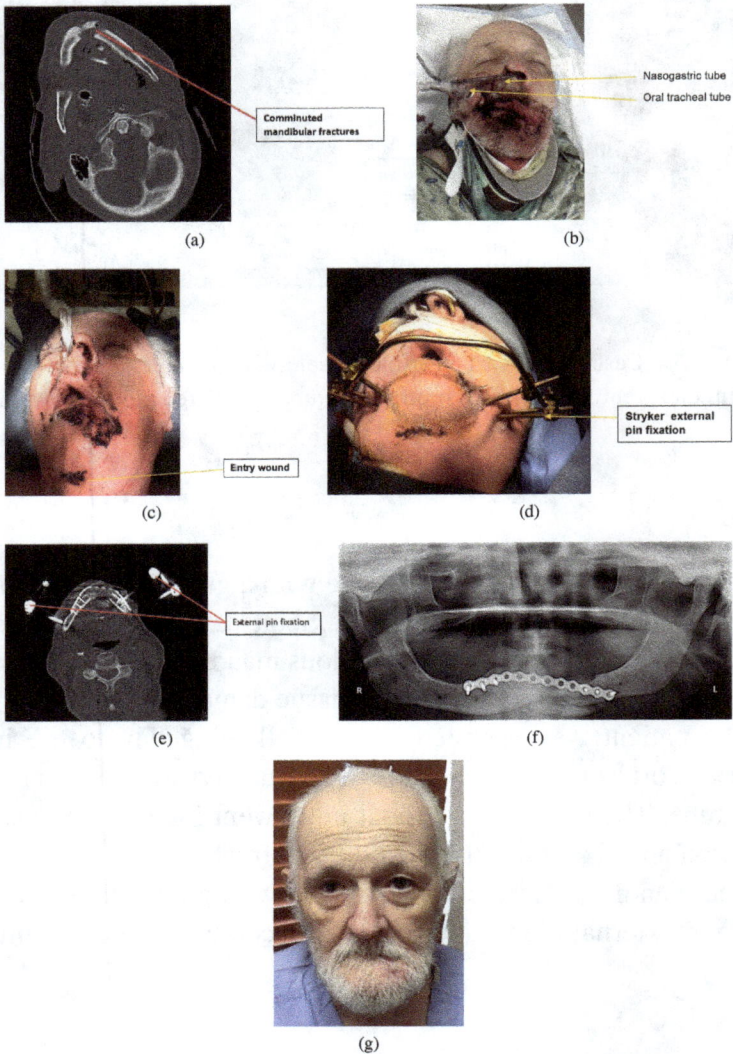

Figure 13.2   Case 2: (a) Axial CT scan shows comminuted mandibular fractures; (b) Patient in the ICU with oral intubation and naso-gastric tube; (c) In the operating theatre, the oral tracheal tube was changed to naso-endotracheal tube for reconstruction of the mandibular fracture; (d) Mandibular reconstruction with external pin fixation and repair of the lip and chin; (e) Post-operative axial CT scan; (f) Two months post-operative orthopantomograph; (g) Patient two months post operatively.

Case 3

A 29-year-old male was shot in the face while standing at a petrol filling station. He sustained a single bullet injury to the right cheek with no underlying fracture, but the soft-tissue injury damaged the right facial nerve (Figure 13.3).

The patient was taken to the operating theatre, and the wound was debrided and the fragmented projectile removed.

In a clean-cut nerve-end injury, the nerve end can be approximated and realigned, then repaired, but in this case, it was not possible to repair the facial nerve due to the extensive damage to the nerve ends caused by the ballistic injuries.

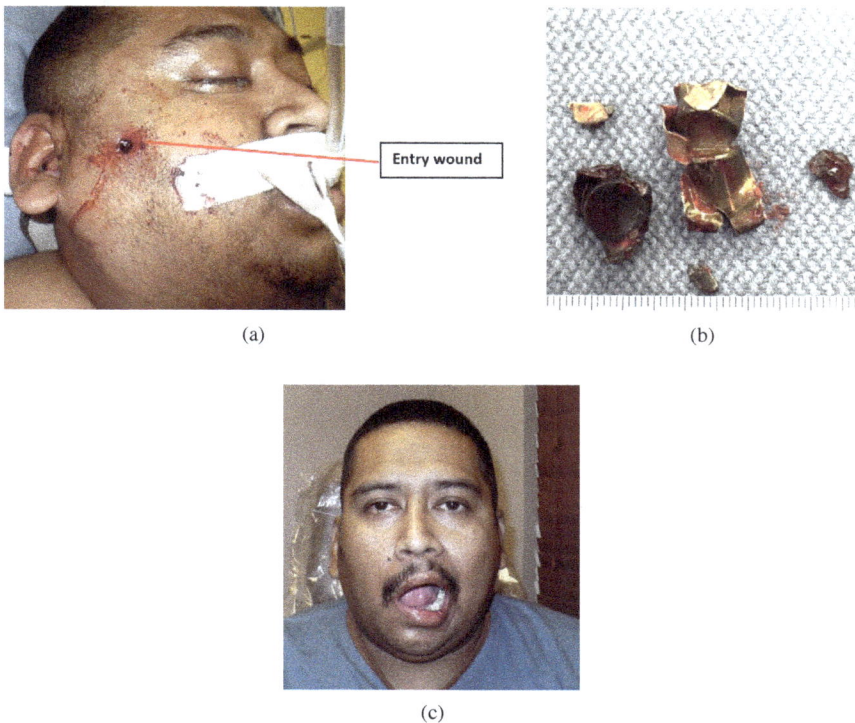

(a)

(b)

(c)

Figure 13.3   Case 3: (a) Patient orally intubated; (b) Fragmented projectile which was removed from the cheek; (c) Two months post surgery with a right lower VII nerve palsy.

Case 4

A 21-year-old male admitted to hospital after being shot with a high-velocity gun. The entry wound was in the right orbit and the bullet exited from the right frontal region. The injury included right frontal lobe herniation, a ruptured right globe, and comminuted frontal and right temporal bone fractures (Figure 13.4).

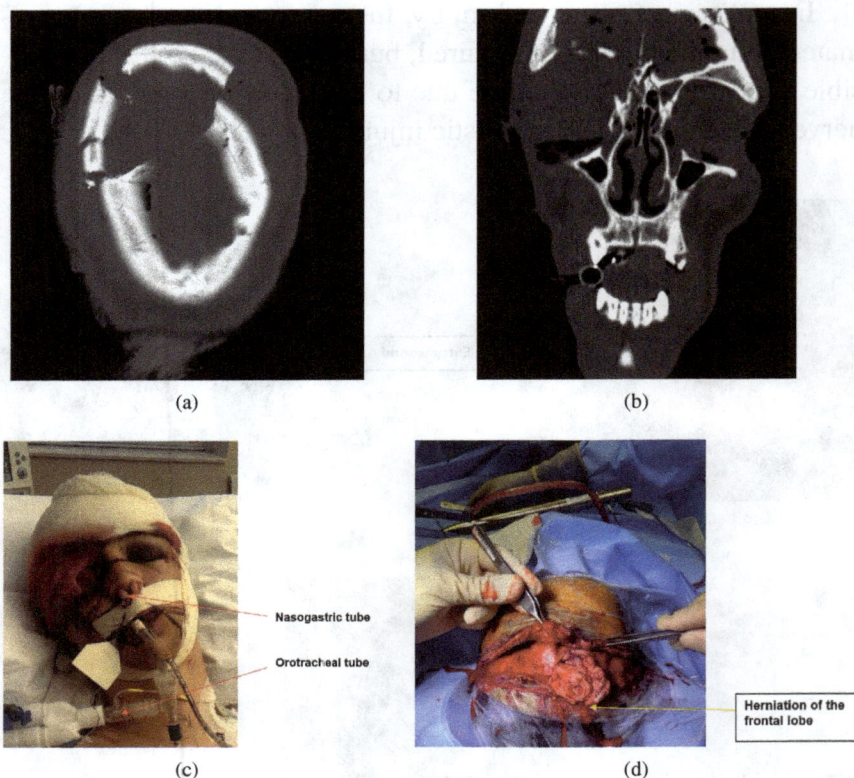

(a)

(b)

Nasogastric tube

Orotracheal tube

Herniation of the frontal lobe

(c)

(d)

Figure 13.4   Case 4: (a) Oblique axial brain CT scan shows right comminuted displaced frontotemporal cranial fractures; (b) Coronal maxillofacial CT scan showing the comminuted right orbital and frontal fractures; (c) Patient intubated on a ventilator in the ICU; (d) Exploration of the right frontal lobe herniation through the exit wound; (e) Miniature plate fixation of the calvarium bone fractures; (f) Axial CT scan showing post craniotomy and fixation of the cranial bones; (g) Patient eight weeks post injury with loss of vision from the right eye.

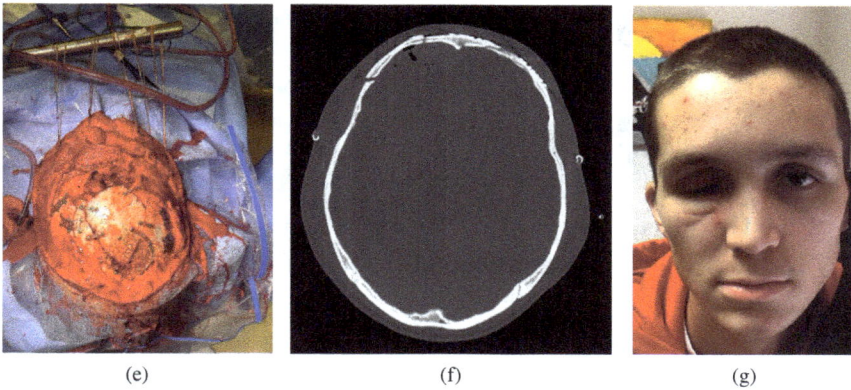

(e) (f) (g)

Figure 13.4 (*Continued*)

The patient underwent an emergency craniotomy, with internal fixation of the calvarium-temporal bone, frontal sinus fractures, and repair of the orbit roof with miniature plates and screws.

Case 5

A 47-year-old male with history of depression was brought to Scottsdale healthcare trauma centre with a shotgun wound to the face in an attempted suicide. He had an emergency cricothyroidotomy and was transported to the trauma centre.

The CT facial scans show comminuted mandible fractures with loss of most of his lower dentition.

The lateral (sagittal) and axial CT scans (Figures 13.5(b) and (c)) show bullet fragments and loss of mandibular continuity.

The patient was taken to the operating theatre and a definitive airway was established with a tracheostomy replacing the cricothyroid tube. Facial hair was removed and the mandibular fracture was stabilised with an internal rigid fixation plate and arch bar. This complex facial laceration was repaired.

Figure 13.5(f) shows the patient five weeks post trauma. The patient's mandible was reconstructed with a bone graft utilising the iliac crest.

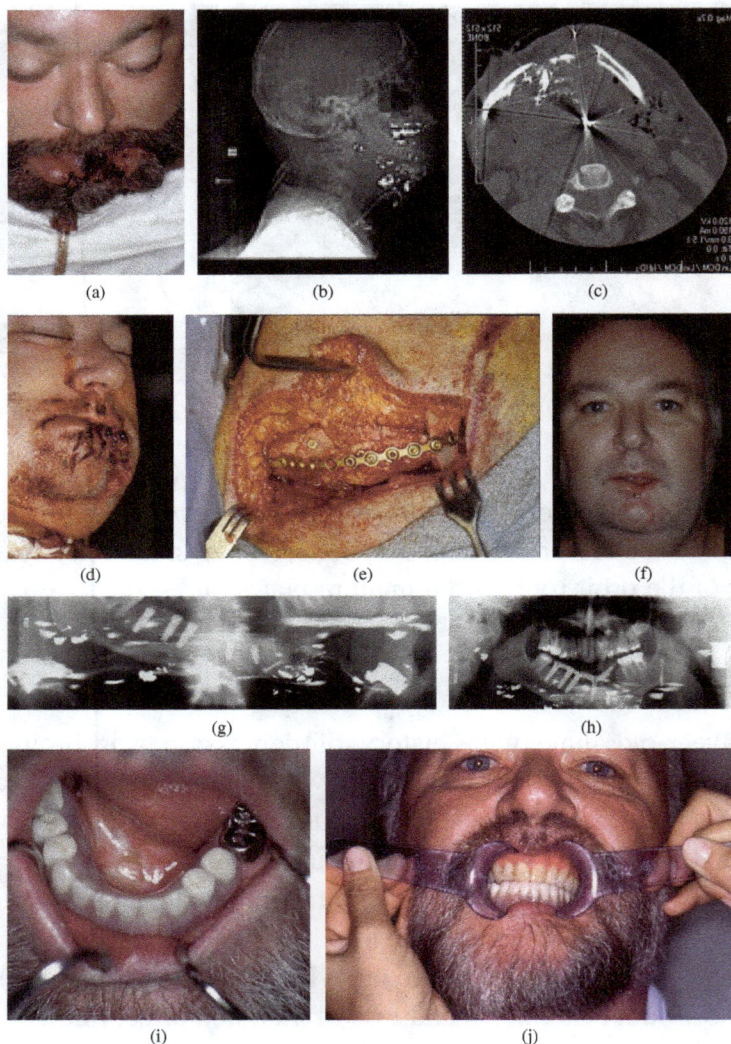

Figure 13.5   Case 5: (a) Emergency cricothyroid tube; (b) Lateral (sagittal) CT scan; (c) Axial CT scan; (d) Extensive lower lip avulsion; (e) Bone graft harvested from the right iliac crest to reconstruct the mandibular defect with rigid fixation; (f) Patient five weeks post trauma; (g) Post-operative endosteal implant placement. The opacities are shrapnel from the shotgun embedded in the soft tissues; (h) Orthopantomograph of the hybrid overdenture. The hybrid lower partial denture was completed 14 months post injury. (i) and (j) Photographs of the patient 14 months post injury.

Six months after the bone graft, five endosteal implants were placed for a future mandibular partial denture reconstruction.

Case 6

A 38-year-old male with a self-inflicted shotgun wound to the face in an attempted suicide. The entry wound was the chin, and the exit wound in the naso-orbital ethmoid region, with severe avulsion of the soft tissue and ruptures of both optic globes. The airway was immediately secured with orotracheal intubation and the patient transported by air to Scottsdale Healthcare trauma centre. The CT scan shows comminuted facial fractures (Figure 13.6(b)). Within 24 hours, a tracheostomy was performed to secure his airway and the wound was closed temporarily. He was medically stabilised to enable definitive reconstructive surgery to be performed later.

This particular case was staged for further surgery to include a cosmetic nasal implant; however, at the request of his wife and due to the loss of his insurance cover, the patient was sent to a hospice for long-term care with no further surgery contemplated.

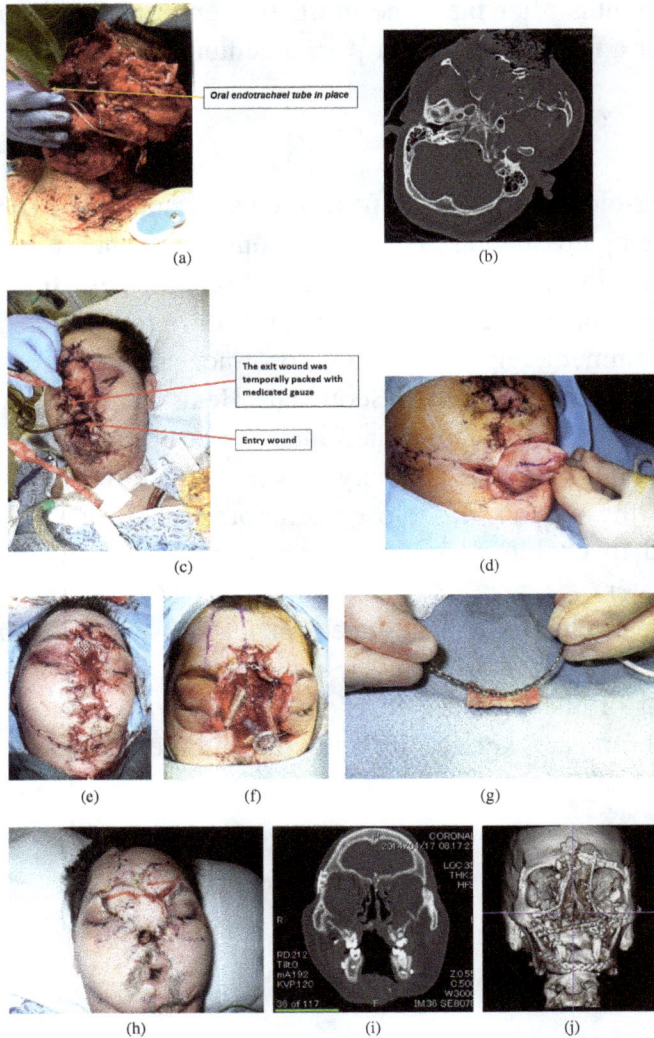

Figure 13.6   Case 6: (a) Patient in the ICU with marked facial avulsion; (b) Immediate CT scan showing comminuted maxillofacial fractures; (c) Immediate post-operative repair of the fractured mandible and suturing of the facial lacerations. The patient lost both optic globes; (d) Closure of the entry wound with a tongue flap and skin graft; (e) Initial wound repair; (f) Reconstruction of both medial orbital walls by rigid fixation with autogenous rib graft; (g) Autogenous rib graft; (h) Ten days after injury, a rotation forehead flap was used to close the missing soft tissue; (i) Post-surgical coronal CT scan; (j) Post-surgical 3-D reconstruction image.

Contrasting Gunshot Wounds from a War Zone (Misrata in 2011)

In contrast to Arizona and similar wealth and peace environments, gunshot wounds observed in war zones can differ in severity, and injury management depends on different factors:

- Type of weapon or the gun i.e. pistol vs. automatic rifle.
- Bullet calibre associated with military-grade weapons (Figure 13.7).
- Distance between the shooter and the victim — in war zones, the distances can be significantly longer.
- Medical facilities available for management.

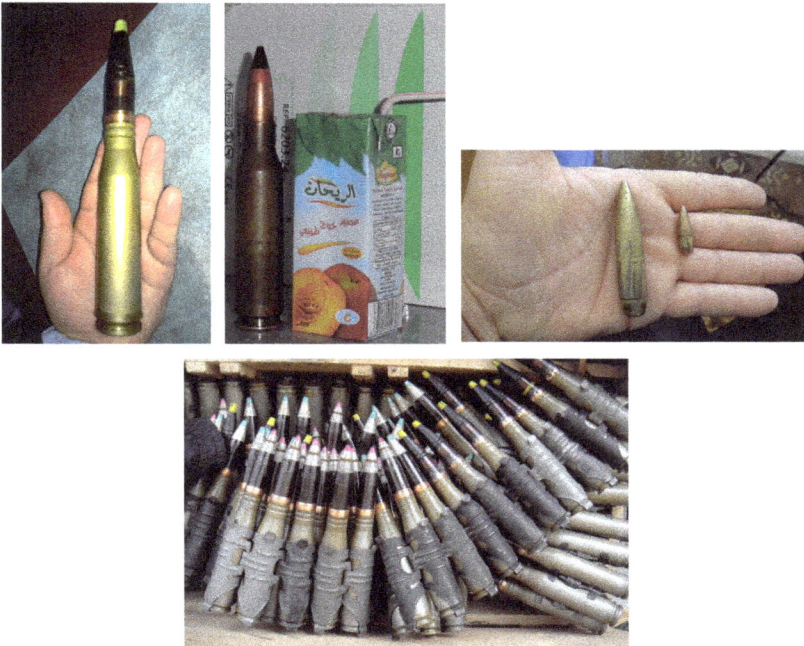

Figure 13.7 Examples of the different sizes of bullets used in the war of Misrata in 2011. These were all found in or with patients. (They are shown with the surgeon's hand for comparison.) The red-tipped bullets are particularly lethal, as they explode on contact.

- Number of casualties, as this significantly affects the mortality, morbidity, and management outcome.

Gunshot injuries in the Arizona cohort are mainly from close range and with short-range guns. In contrast, in a war zone, gunshots can be from much greater distances and with types of ammunition that are intended to cause maximum damage. As such, these factors can dictate the impact of the bullet. Soft-tissue injuries will always occur; however, the impact with the bone can result in bone shattering, breaking, or an impact where the bullet changes direction, all of which depends on the bullet, gun, and distance. Figure 13.8 shows a long-distance bullet wound to the right side of the face. Due to the long distance, the bullet changed direction in the soft tissue and had to be removed intraorally rather than via the original entry wound.

In Figure 13.9, the bullet ended in the scalp but failed to go through the hard bone of the skull allowing for easy removal of the bullet.

This bullet in Figure 13.10 hit the mandibular bone through the soft tissue and changed its direction to the base of the neck, where it was located by the surgeon.

In some cases, the pathway of the bullet is ambiguous. In Figure 13.11, the bullet entered above the clavicle, travelled through the soft tissue to end up sublingual.

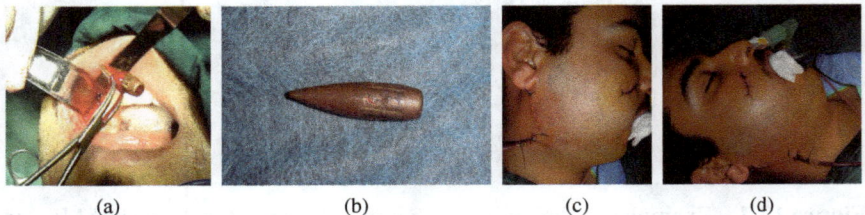

(a)   (b)   (c)   (d)

Figure 13.8   (a–d) Long-distance bullet wound.

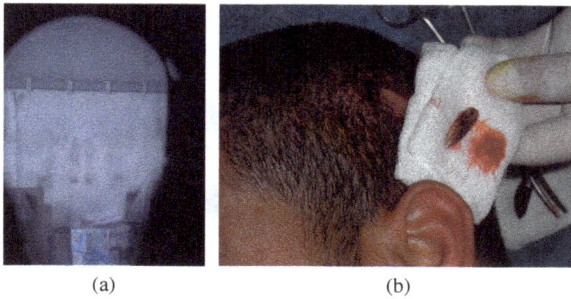

Figure 13.9   (a) and (b) Easily removed bullet.

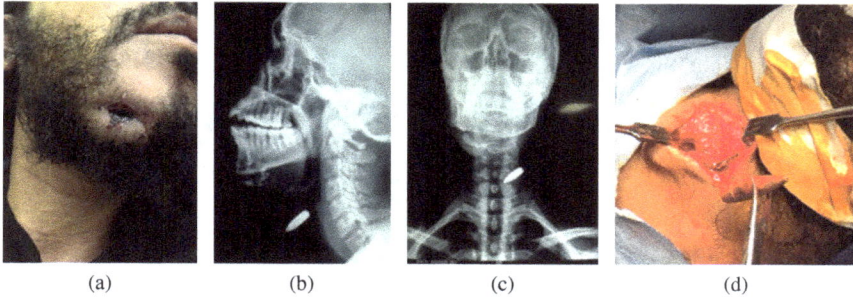

Figure 13.10   (a–d) Bullet changed direction after entry.

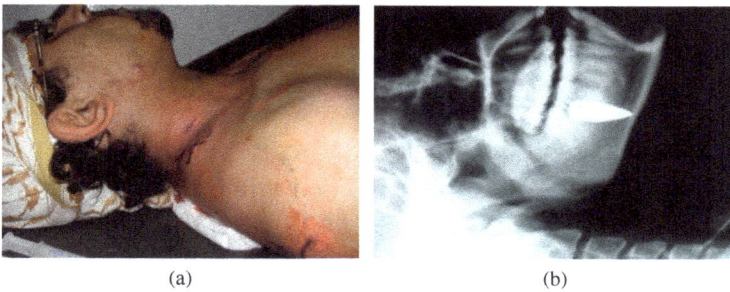

Figure 13.11   (a) and (b).

The injuries in Figure 13.12 were inflicted by a sniper rifle which is an advanced gun with a specific bullet type designed for maximum damage. Most commonly, the destruction is significant and the bullet

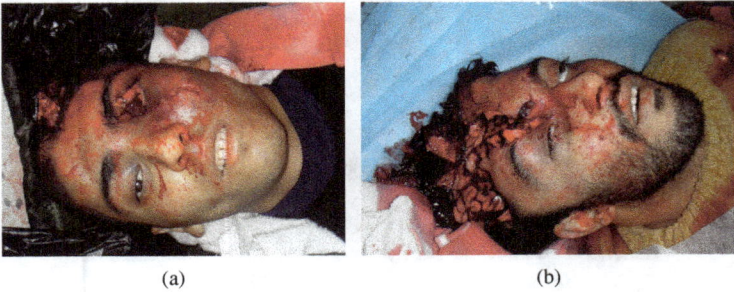

(a)   (b)

Figure 13.12   (a) and (b) Sniper shots.

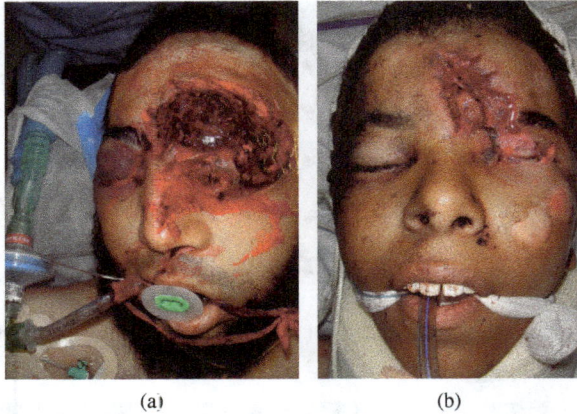

(a)   (b)

Figure 13.13   (a) and (b) Sniper-fire victims who survived their injuries.

hits vital structures in the craniofacial region, so patients are highly unlikely to survive. These patients died while being transported to the hospital. The patients in Figure 13.13 survived.

Conclusion

Protection of the soft-tissue envelope must be secured for reconstruction of the skeletal foundation as soon as the patient is medically stable. This will reduce scar contracture and the loss of adequate facial projection.

These cases clearly show that gun violence, both suicide and assault, are a major public health issue in the US from social and economic points of view. The consequences affect entire families and communities. The permanent damage ranges from functional and cosmetic deformity to financial difficulties for the injured patient and their family due to high healthcare costs.

Reference

1. Gun Violence Archive. Past summary ledgers 2014–2019. n.d.-a. https://www.gunviolencearchive.org/past-tolls.

Index

www.ingramcontent.com/pod-product-compliance
Lightning Source LLC
Chambersburg PA
CBHW050550190326
41458CB00007B/1987

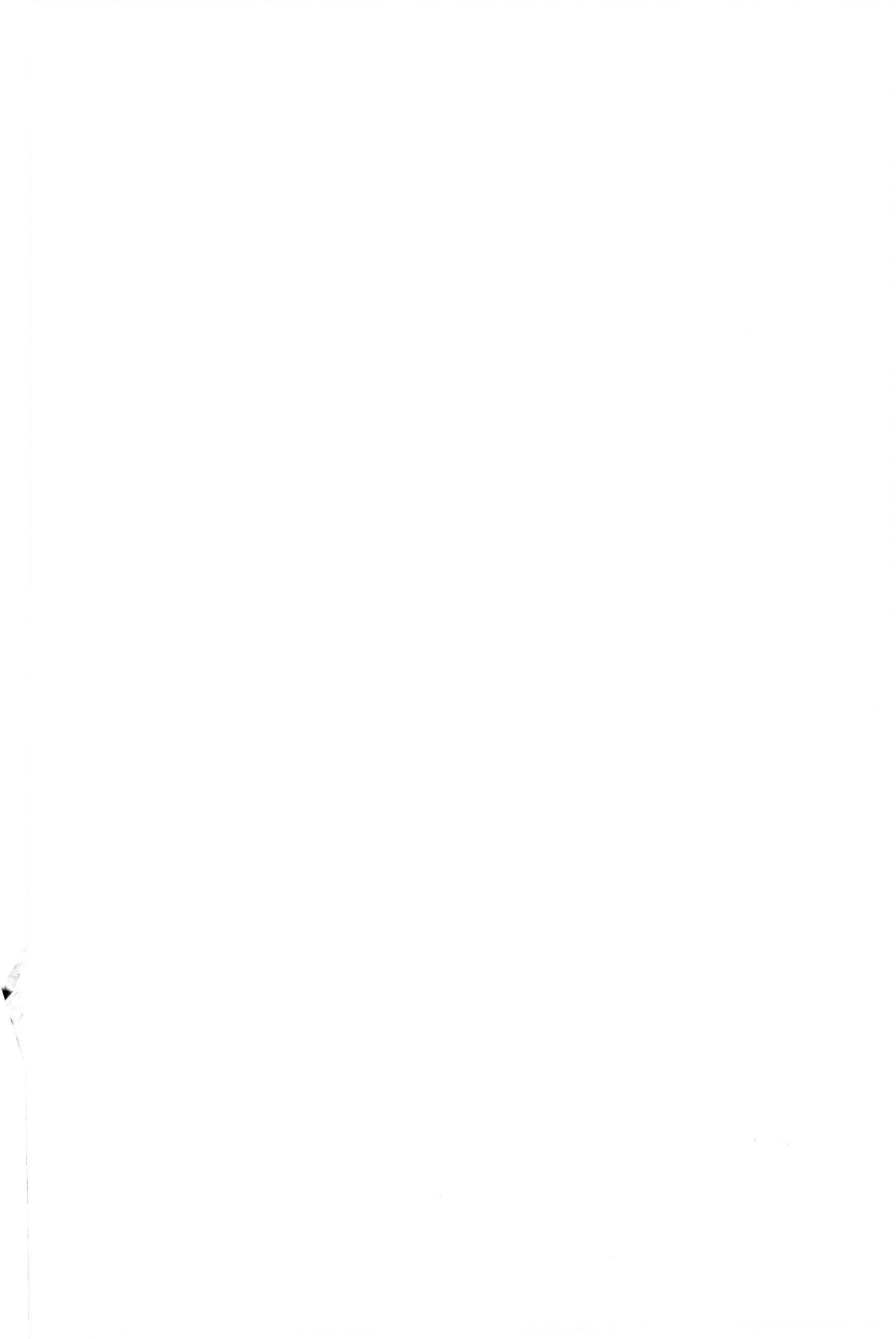